Candida

A NATURAL APPROACH

Candida

A NATURAL APPROACH

Shirley Trickett
Karen Brody

Ulysses Press  Berkeley, CA
1999

Published by: Ulysses Press
           P.O. Box 3440
           Berkeley, CA 94703-3440

Library of Congress Catalog Card Number: 98-85069
ISBN: 1-56975-153-6

First published in the United Kingdom as *Coping With Candida* and *The Candida Diet Book* by Sheldon Press

Printed in Canada by Transcontinental Printing

10 9 8 7 6 5 4 3 2 1

Editor: Mark Woodworth
Cover Design: Leslie Henriques
Cover Illustration: "Woman #2," Diana Ong/SuperStock Fine Arts
Editorial and production staff: Steven Schwartz, Natasha Lay,
   Lily Chou, David Wells
Indexer: Sayre Van Young

"Nursing Mothers" section written by Heather Welford

Distributed in the United States by Publishers Group West
and in Canada by Raincoast Books

All names and identifying characteristics of real persons have been changed in the text to protect their confidentiality.

Contents

Note from the Publisher

This book has been written and published strictly for informational purposes, and in no way should it be used as a substitute for consultation with your medical doctor or health care professional. All facts in this book came from medical files, clinical journals, scientific publications, personal interviews, published trade books, self-published materials by experts, magazine articles, and the personal-practice experiences of the authorities quoted or sources cited. You should not consider educational material herein to be the practice of medicine or to replace consultation with a physician or other medical practitioner. The author and publisher are providing you with information in this work so that you can have the knowledge and can choose, at your own risk, to act on that knowledge. The author and publisher also urge all readers to be aware of their health status and to consult health professionals before beginning any health program, including changes in dietary habits.

PART I

By Shirley Trickett

Coping With Candida

Although I believe in empowerment, and am a self-help teacher working in the field of complementary medicine, I still have one foot in the other camp (traditional medicine) and believe self-diagnosis is dangerous. Therefore, it is important for you to consult with a doctor, describing your symptoms to a professional, before you embark on this or any other self-help program.

CHAPTER ONE

The Candida Question

Candida albicans—why write a book on an organism that is present in the gut of nearly every individual soon after birth, a yeast commonly thought to be responsible for little more than irritating skin rashes or infections of the mouth or vagina? The answer is that 20th-century living is slowly changing the human immune system. The environment, prescribed drugs (including the Pill), street drugs, the ever-increasing consumption of alcohol, junk food, additives, sugar, and the pace of modern living all have had a negative impact on our immune systems. And, a healthy gut is a key factor in maintaining the immune system. The intestines need to be like a balanced ecological system; they need an environment where there are enough "good" bacteria to attack harmful bacteria, keeping the growth of fungus (yeasts) at bay.

What an Overgrowth of Candida Can Do

When candida or other harmful yeasts proliferate, they block the sites of the bowel where the enzymes necessary for the breakdown of food inhabit. This results in poor digestion, food intolerance, bloating, and altered bowel habits. An overgrowth of candida in the colon can also inhibit the absorption of essential nutrients, creating vitamin and mineral deficiencies. In addition, the vitamins normally manufactured in the bowel cannot be produced when the colon is in this state, and thus the problem is compounded.

When there is a proliferation of candida it can change from its simple form, which looks like a microscopic fried egg, to a complicated invasive form which grows tentacles that can penetrate the bowel wall. This not only allows the toxins produced by candida to circulate, but also gives the organism transportation to other parts of the body where infections can arise, resulting in any of the following symptoms:

- chronic fatigue
- food intolerance
- PMS
- sinus infections
- ear infections
- food cravings
- chronic cystitis
- yeast and other vaginal infections
- hormonal imbalance
- fluid retention
- sore throats
- inflammation of the digestive tract
- infections of the penis and scrotum
- chest problems
- skin problems
- allergies
- nail-bed infections
- muscle and joint pains

- athlete's foot

- being underweight

- obesity and an inability to lose weight on a low-calorie diet

The toxins from candida can also cause severe psychological symptoms such as agitation, mood swings, anxiety, insomnia, and depression.

The Medical Argument

Because of a general lack of awareness about candida, and the diversity of symptoms, some of which could be interpreted as hypochondriasis, the long-term candida sufferer often endures endless tests without the condition ever being diagnosed. If treatment is given it is often in the form of antibiotics, which only aggravate the symptoms. Or more than likely the patient is told, "This is only your nerves—why not take a vacation?"

Some doctors believe there is no foundation for chronic candidiasis. Others believe the abdominal symptoms may be the result of fermentation in the gut. (Fermentation, as any amateur brewer knows, needs yeast!) Two physicians, O. C. Truss and William Crook, believe that candida can cause widespread problems in the body and have done much to raise "candida consciousness," both in the medical profession and among sufferers. Generally, however, real understanding of the ever-growing fungal problem is in its infancy.

My experience leads me to believe that any condition that the average doctor has not studied in medical school does not exist in his or her mind. In saying that, please do not think I do not respect the medical profession. I have met many doctors who are open-minded, who use their own intuitive knowledge, and who let their patients fully express their intuitive feelings about their own bodies before they reach for the prescription pad. I am not anti-drug, but I am very much against some of the lethal pharmacological cocktails commonly prescribed in these pills-for-all-ills days. I am also concerned about the endless repeat prescriptions for "safe" drugs, such as medications for gastric ulcers. I have seen too many prescribed-drug-damaged people, and, in the case of candida, I have seen too many people who face their doctors with a chronic condition that is a result of drug treatments.

What Is Fungus?

The fungi family include molds, mushrooms, yeasts, and rusts. They are simple plants that lack chlorophyll and are either parasitic, living off live matter, or saprophytic, living off dead matter.

Fungus consists of a mass of fine threads from which branches grow upward. Spores are released from spore cases at the end of each branch. These grow into a new "individual" and can be carried by the wind. Fungi are all around us: in our bodies, in the soil, and in the air. Some are helpful to us for digestion, baking, brewing, and producing antibiotics; others are responsible for disease in humans, animals, and plants.

Yeasts are single-cell organisms that reproduce by budding (the formation of a small outgrowth that grows and breaks off) and possess enzymes capable of converting sugar into ethanol (alcohol). This process, *fermentation*, causes the release of carbon dioxide. (In breadmaking, the dough "rises" because of this gas.) Other products of fermentation include citric acid, oxalic acid, and butyric acid (see page 26). These acids are formed by certain bacteria.

Is It Only Candida that Causes Problems?

No. The fungi that cause infections are too numerous to mention, but for the purpose of this book the term fungus is used except where the yeast *Candida albicans* is known to be the culprit. If the body is weakened by an overgrowth of candida in the bowel other fungi can intrude, and the virulence of some of the harmful bacteria can also increase.

What Can I Do to Cope with Fungal Infections?

- Clean the colon
- Stop feeding the fungus through a proper diet
- Kill the fungus, with drug or nondrug antifungal agents
- Replace with good bacteria in the gut using probiotics
- Boost the immune system with nutritional supplements
- Boost the immune system by taking care of your general health

CHAPTER TWO

The Likely Candidates

As I have mentioned before, there is an increase in fungal infections in the general population because of modern living. Predisposing factors that make some people particularly vulnerable are listed below:

- any debilitating illness that weakens the immune system, such as flu, pneumonia, cancer, or AIDS. (When the body already has more work than it can cope with, it cannot be vigilant enough to keep organisms in the gut under control. In addition, immunosuppressant drugs, often vital in life-threatening diseases, encourage the body to play host to candida and other fungi. Adequate nutrition and supplements can prevent fungal overgrowth in seriously ill patients and improve their prognosis and quality of life.)

- frequent treatment with antibiotics in the present or past

- using contraceptive pills

- taking various prescribed medications (or, more commonly, after withdrawal from them); for example: steroids, ulcer drugs, tranquilizers and sleeping pills, long-term antacids

- malnutrition from lack of vitamins and minerals and/or a highly refined carbohydrate diet or junk food
- stress
- endocrine disorders, diabetes
- genetic inability to cope with candida or carbohydrates
- anemia
- after any surgery, particularly abdominal surgery
- bowel infections, gastroenteritis
- damage to the urinary tract through catheterization
- hormonal imbalance: the premenstrual phase, pregnancy, menopause
- multiple pregnancies
- impairing the immune system through lack of exercise, fresh air, or working in a polluted environment
- street drugs
- alcohol
- lack of hydrochloric acid
- infection from a sexual partner
- a medical history of the following:
  —repeated bacterial infections
  —hyperactivity as a child
  —allergies
  —swollen painful joints for no apparent cause
  —oral thrush
  —mouth ulcers
  —chronic sinusitis
  —erratic vision, including spots before the eyes

—vaginal yeast infections

—vulval itching

—itchy rectum or anus

—cystitis-like symptoms

—severe PMS

—unexplained mild rise in body temperature

—jock itch

—athlete's foot, ringworm, psoriasis, nail-bed infections (a different organism but often associated with candida), acne

—craving for sweet or yeast-containing foods

—feeling worse after consuming refined carbohydrates, alcohol, cheese, citrus juice, vitamin B or vitamin C tablets, soft drinks containing citric acid

—abdominal distention, breathing problems, or any other symptoms associated with the proximity to certain chemicals

—gas, bloating, cramps, constipation, diarrhea

—being weather-sensitive, i.e., worse in humid or wet weather

—feeling worse in musty or moldy places

—irritability, confused thinking, poor memory, being spaced out, feeling drunk without alcohol, experiencing depression

Many people say, "But I haven't had a yeast infection for years." If your body has been coping with an overgrowth of candida for some time it may no longer be responding with an acute infection; it has become tolerant to the effects of the organism.

Though not an invitation to self-diagnose, I have provided you with some of the information you need to know to determine whether or not candida could be a problem. I have opened up an opportunity for you to look for other avenues of help when you have been told that there is no apparent reason for your problems, or that your problems are "just nerves."

"Brain" Symptoms

As noted before, in chronic sufferers the body stops reacting with acute symptoms. What follows can be classified as what I call "brain" symptoms—vague feelings such as those that resemble having a permanent hangover or feeling exhausted without being able to pinpoint specific problems. Such people often say they feel poisoned, depressed, and have no interest in anything.

The waste products of candida can escape from the bowel into the bloodstream and "poison" the brain. When the biochemistry of the brain is seriously affected it gives rise to psychological symptoms. In this instance, however, the symptoms have their foundation in a physical cause. It is therefore useless to treat the "brain" symptoms of candidiasis—which can range from feelings of hopelessness, irritability, confusion, anxiety, and depression to a schizophrenic-like state—with tranquilizers, antidepressants, or psychotherapy. (However, psychotherapy can often be useful because such sufferers may have life problems because of their condition, but this must be as an adjunct to anti-candida treatment.)

How Do You Know It's Not Just Depression?

It is true that many of the above symptoms appear in any depressive state and many depressed people feel that there is something physically wrong with them. But in cases where there is any significant history, particularly if there are allergies, and especially where the person has failed to respond to antidepressants, it is worth trying the anti-candida approach.

Systemic Candidiasis

Lisa had been ill for four years. After a period of prolonged stress she developed recurrent vaginal infections, cystitis, and severe premenstrual tension. These problems were all new to her and she became increasingly anxious and depressed. Her boyfriend and colleagues began to lose patience with her. She feared her job was in jeopardy. She had formerly enjoyed her work, but particularly when she was premenstrual, she became very anxious about going to the office because she reacted so explosively to events that would previously have merely caused her to feel mildly irritated. Visits to the doctor resulted in prescriptions for cream for the vaginal infection and antibiotics for the cystitis. She was also urged to stop worrying.

Although she was losing weight, her abdomen grew alarmingly in size; she could not fasten her skirts. This coincided with changed bowel habits: alternating bouts of constipation and diarrhea. Even when her stool was loose, she felt "gassy" and never felt as if she had cleared her bowel. This was diagnosed as Irritable Bowel Syndrome, which her doctor said was due to nerves. He suggested a high-fiber diet and again to stop worrying.

When the next set of symptoms arrived two months later, Lisa saw another doctor in the practice. She complained of swelling inside her nose, aching sinuses, and a dry cough. She also mentioned she felt ill when she ate certain foods and when she was near certain chemicals, all symptoms associated with food intolerance. In addition, she had palpitations, restlessness, depression, and hives. The effect of the chemical intolerance was a feeling of being "spaced out"—with head-aches and inability to concentrate. Also, the smells in her new car and from the photocopier at work seemed to affect her in particular.

She left the office with a prescription for a nasal spray and antihista-mines. Both helped a little but she was still dissatisfied. She began reading health magazines and books and was delighted when she read an article in a newspaper by a woman who had an identical experience to her own. Armed with information on systemic fungal infections she saw yet another doctor in the practice. To her surprise and delight he agreed candida could be the problem and prescribed Nystatin. Lisa put herself on a strict anti-candida diet and for the first three weeks she still felt poorly. New symptoms developed that she rightly credited to "die off." (See page 100.) The symptoms included a slight temperature, feelings of confusion, and muscle and joint pains. As these cleared she made steady progress; all the symptoms she had suffered for years just seemed to fade away. Friends com-mented on her appearance: her face regained its normal contours (it had been bloated) and was free from the bumps under the skin and dryness that had contributed to her misery over the years.

Lisa's story illustrates the diverse nature of chronic candidiasis, how seriously the hormone balance can be upset by the condition, and also how using Nystatin can restore immune competence by killing the candida, allowing the body to cope with infections in other sites. Presumably this happens when toxins from the candida and the undigested particles of protein have stopped "leaking" from the infected bowel.

Candida and Women

It is understandable that there is a higher incidence of candidiasis in women than in men. Oral contraceptives and hormonal influences play a major role. In addition, the close proximity of the perineum (the area between the anus and the vagina), and the relatively short length of the urethra (the tube leading to the bladder), could account for women having more acute infections. (Nevertheless, men are by no means immune from candidiasis and the numbers of sufferers are increasing. When an overgrowth is established in the bowel, men suffer the same digestive problems, allergies, and "brain" symptoms as do women.)

The Premenstrual Phase and Candida

Any hormonal disturbance can trigger an acute attack of candida. Oral contraceptives have been shown to markedly increase the vaginal glucose content, thus providing a good "food" supply for the candida. In the premenstrual phase, during pregnancy, and during steroid medication the delicate acid/alkaline balance of the vaginal secretions is also altered, encouraging fungal growth.

Menopause and Candida

During menopause the vagina often loses its natural lubrication and becomes dry and cracked. This condition is called *atrophic vaginitis* and is caused by a decrease in estrogen levels. When the tender mucus membrane of the vagina is torn, candida easily gains entry. Estrogen creams are often prescribed for this problem, or a simple lubricant such as KY jelly or Astroglide is suggested.

In addition, there are natural ways of increasing estrogen levels. It is noted that Japanese women have fewer symptoms of menopause than Western women. This may be due to that fact that they consume more phytoestrogens (plant estrogens). Phytoestrogens are found in soy beans, tofu, miso, dates, flaxseed, and pomegranates. These foods act like those estrogens naturally produced in the body. There are a number of books available, including *Menopause, Naturally* by Sadga Greenwood (Volcano Press), with helpful information about natural hormone replacement. (See "Further Reading" at the back of the book.)

Vaginal Yeast Infections

One in every two women are afflicted with vaginal yeast infections at one time or another. Many are plagued by recurring infections, which are most frequent between the ages of 16 and 35. These repeated infections, which often go hand-in-hand with cystitis, can make life miserable. Acute attacks are characterized by itching and soreness of the vagina and labia, accompanied by a creamy white or yellow discharge that can have a cheesy odor.

(Vaginitis caused by the *gardnerella* bacteria produces a grayish, frothy discharge that can be mistaken for a yeast infection. If you have an infection that does not respond to anti-candida treatment you might have gardnerella and would need to see your doctor for medication. Women with gardnerella who are prone to yeast infections may have a combined infection necessitating both antibacterial and antifungal treatment. The infection caused by the parasite *trichomonas vaginalis* is also sometimes confused with yeast infection. The symptoms are similar but the discharge is usually darker and the smell stronger. A doctor will be needed to prescribe medication for this condition as well.)

For nondrug preparations that are effective against fungal, bacterial, and parasitic infections see pages 50–55.

An isolated attack of yeast infection that clears quickly with treatment is of no consequence. The fungus may have gained entry because of some slight injury to the vaginal tissue, either by vigorous sexual intercourse, a tampon, clothes chafing, or horseback riding. Long hot hours sitting while traveling, particularly in nylon underwear or tight jeans, can also precipitate an attack. If, however, you are having regular infections, even if they do clear with over-the-counter creams, you should investigate why this is happening. Look at the predisposing factors:

- How stressed are you?
- Is your immune system working well?
- Do you have a healthy diet?
- Is your partner reinfecting you?

Women with a reservoir of candida in the bowel or deep in the vagina are more likely to suffer repeated attacks of yeast infections, although some women with chronic candidiasis stop reacting with acute attacks. It is common for a chronic candida sufferer to say, "Oh yes, I had recurrent yeast infections for years but I don't get them now." It is important for women who have repeated attacks of yeast infections to be treated with more than topical medications since candida can spread to the reproductive organs and cause pelvic pain.

Treatment for Vaginal Yeast Infections

Diflucan (fluconazole) pessaries or creams, Femstat (butoconazole nitrate), or Terazol (terconazole) are the medications generally prescribed by doctors. Over-the-counter medications include Monistat 7 (miconazole nitrate) and Gyne-Lotrimin (clotrimazole), and can be bought at any pharmacy.

A more natural approach, live plain yogurt is soothing and can clear up a mild attack. Douching twice daily with ten drops of tea tree oil (see pages 59–60) in a pint of warm water or using tea tree cream can also be very effective. Tea tree has a mild local anesthetic effect that is very helpful for relieving itching and soreness. Garlic douches, two crushed cloves in a pint of warm water, can also bring relief. In Britain, Cervagyn vaginal cream, a blend of acidophilus with emollients derived from vegetable oils that helps maintain normal vaginal flora and penetrates deeply into the vaginal tissue, is available. It has been shown to be a very effective product. It is available in a tube with an applicator from BioCare (see "Useful Addresses").

HYGIENE

After a bowel movement clean yourself from the vagina toward the anus, and if possible wash the area in cool water. Avoid long, hot baths. Showers are preferable or take a warm bath with ten drops of tea tree oil. Juniper and sandalwood oils are also helpful for cystitis—for more information on essential oils see page 58.

Empty the bladder and douche with either cool water or one of the suggested solutions after sexual intercourse. Men can be symptom-free but still carry candida so it is important for them to pay strict attention to hygiene and to be treated concurrently with their partner if they have an infection.

CLOTHING

Warm, damp conditions encourage yeast infections so avoid nylon underwear, pantyhose, and tight jeans. Stockings are the obvious choice, but if you prefer pantyhose, buy the ones with cotton crotches. Since underwear harbors yeast spores, wear only white cotton underwear and buy a larger size than usual. They invariably shrink during vigorous laundering. Avoid using wash cloths. To save having to launder a large towel after use, dry the vaginal area with a wash cloth or small towel and disinfect it along with your underwear. Alternatively, you could dry the area with toilet tissue (preferably unbleached). When laundering, avoid harsh biological detergents. Old-fashioned boiling in plain water is cheap and safe, or you could scrub the crotch with soap and pour boiling water over it. Treat the crotch of swimwear in the same way, or allow it to dry in the sun. Soaking underwear in a solution of tea tree oil and then washing it with the rest of your laundry is another way to treat your clothing.

Women, Candidiasis, and the Effects on the Brain

When sufferers present their symptoms of lethargy, anxiety, or depression to their doctors they are often told it's only nerves, or their symptoms are attributed to their hormones. It's PMS; it's PMS extending over more of the month now that you are past 35; it's menopause. Undoubtedly, part of the story, as we have seen, can be attributed to hormones, but what about the other effects? And why do these women fail to respond to tranquilizers, antidepressants, and treatments for hormonal problems? Why do they only recover when they acquire knowledge of candidiasis and act on it? Misdiagnosis in women causes frustration, loss of confidence, and because of this, psychological problems are superimposed on the existing physiological manifestations of altered brain chemistry. When a woman starts to feel better with anti-candida treatment there may be angry tears: "I knew it was something in my body that was causing this; why didn't the doctor listen to me?"

Candida and Mothers and Babies

Heather Welford, a writer and breastfeeding counselor notes that candida can affect the early weeks and months of your baby's life and bring pain and discomfort to one of motherhood's most pleasurable and rewarding experiences—breastfeeding. Candida on the nipples, and in the breast itself, can cause soreness, both during and between feeding. It can be bad enough to make even the most dedicated and motivated breastfeeder turn to the bottle out of desperation. Babies, too, can get painful yeast infections on their bottoms and in their genital area. They can also have candida in the mouth (thrush), and this may mean it's painful to suck on a breast or bottle.

Thrush and Feeding

When a breastfeeding mother complains of soreness, breastfeeding counselors and professional lactation specialists are usually well aware that thrush could be the reason, but many general practitioners are still unaware of the possibility. Mothers are sometimes told to stop nursing or they're given creams and sprays that have no effect on the problem, and may make it even worse.

Breastfeeding provides an ideal environment for candida to flourish, especially here in the West, where breasts might be covered for most of the time with a hot, sweaty, synthetic bra, maybe with a plastic-backed breastpad tucked inside for good measure.

In addition, many new mothers and babies are prescribed antibiotics for postnatal infections contracted in the hospital. Doctors may also prescribe antibiotics as a routine preventive measure to mothers who have had a cesarean section (over 20 percent of deliveries in the U.S. are cesareans) and, as mentioned before, antibiotics create conditions suitable for the overgrowth of candida.

If either you or your baby has a yeast infection or thrush, breastfeeding can mean you pass it back and forth between you. Bottle-fed babies can get thrush in their mouths, too, as can babies who use pacifiers.

Sore Bottoms

Disposable diapers keep your baby's bottom warm and moist—again an ideal condition for yeast infections. Candida can affect the anus, the buttocks, the genitals, and the top of the legs as well.

Symptoms

You may have sore, red, raw, or itchy nipples. Sometimes the skin seems to flake away. The nipples are tender between feedings, and it can be very painful when the baby latches on. (If you've been sore since the very beginning of nursing then poor positioning—with your baby sucking on the end of your nipples instead of being well latched on to the breast—is a more likely cause of discomfort than thrush. Of course, you can get thrush on top of soreness caused by poor positioning; if you're pretty sure your positioning is correct and you still don't heal, suspect candida.)

You may also get intense stabbing or shooting pains in the breast, most acute when the baby is actually feeding or shortly afterward. The pain tends to radiate out from the nipple and may indicate that there is thrush in the breast milk ducts, or in the areas of the breast surrounding the ducts. It is possible to get this pain without any soreness on the nipples.

If your baby is affected by thrush he or she may have a red shiny patchy rash on his or her genital area that doesn't go away with the usual remedies for diaper rash (exposing the bottom to the air or application of diaper rash cream and frequent diaper changes). The effects can be painful and cause your baby some distress. However, even quite dramatic looking symptoms may not produce any soreness.

Oral thrush shows up as whitish deposits in your baby's mouth: on the tongue, the inside of the cheeks, and the gums. A few babies show some reluctance to feed and cry when they suck. However, some babies with thrush don't show any symptoms. It is reasonable to assume that if you have it and you're breastfeeding, then your baby has it too.

Treatment

- Discard all the nipples and pacifiers you're using and buy new ones (sterilize them before use). The same goes for any nipple shields. Shields are sometimes used to protect sore nipples but they can make the problem worse, not better. Ask for help in positioning your baby on your breast so you no longer need a shield.

- Wear a cotton bra and change your breastpads often. Use non-plastic backed ones.

- See your doctor for antifungal medication and insist on treatment for both you and your baby if you're breastfeeding. Persistent candida can take a couple of weeks or more to clear, though you should see an improvement in a few days.

- Make sure you pay extra attention to family hygiene, with separate washcloths and towels for each of you. Check other members of the family for candida, especially your sexual partner.

- If the yeast infection persists, check your diet (see page 61) and try some of the suggestions in Chapter Seven.

Trisha had been nursing her baby Joshua for nine weeks with no problems at all. Then she developed sore nipples. She described them as "feeling raw." Nursing was very painful, and her nipples were tender between feedings, as well. Her doctor could give no explanation as to why she should develop the soreness after so many weeks of problem-free nursing and prescribed lanolin cream to soothe her nipples. This, if anything, made the problem worse.

By chance, Trisha met a breastfeeding counselor at a friend's house. The counselor said the problem could be caused by candida, and this seemed even more likely when Trisha reported a recent bout with a vaginal yeast infection that had started after a course of antibiotics for an infection.

Trisha's doctor was willing to consider this diagnosis, and when Trisha went back he prescribed two separate antifungal preparations, one for her and one for Joshua. In a few days the soreness had gone.

Candida and Men

Men going to the doctor with intestinal candida are more likely to be told they are suffering from diverticulosis or stress than from candida. The chronic symptom picture in men is identical to that of women— that is to say, doctors see the patient as having the same "neurotic" symptoms as women (lethargy and ill temper). The only differences are obvious biological ones (hormone imbalances) as well as more alcohol-related candida and chemical intolerance due to exposure in the workplace. Men suffer just as much from digestive problems and food allergies, in fact probably more. The case history on page 42 describes the devastation systemic candidiasis can cause in a man's life and the story is by no means unusual.

Acute Attacks

Infection around the genitals—better known as "jock itch"— is common in men with candida. Candida in men often manifests itself as NSU (nonspecific urethritis), an inflammation of the urethra. This problem needs medical attention because it can lead to the more serious condition called Reiter's syndrome, which consists of arthritis, urethritis, conjunctivitis, and sometimes fever and rashes. If the penis is inflamed it is more likely to be a combined bacterial and fungal infection.

Other conditions caused by yeast infections include severe acne and athlete's foot. (Men tend to suffer more from athlete's foot than do women.) If the athlete's foot persists after following strict hygiene, local antifungal treatment, wearing cotton socks, airing shoes, and not wearing the same pair of shoes every day, your general health may be impaired or there could be an overgrowth of candida in the bowel.

Contact Dermatitis/Candida

Contact dermatitis from belt buckles, metal on jeans, or from laundry detergent is often complicated by fungal infections and can be very persistent. If your efforts at finding the offending material and using an antifungal cream fail it is advisable to see your doctor.

Avoid pants made from synthetic materials, tight jeans, nylon underwear, and briefs (even cotton ones). Boxer shorts allow better circulation.

Other Causes of Candida in Men

Because of raised glucose levels in the blood, diabetic men are more prone to fungal infections. Their perspiration can often smell yeasty.

Heavy drinking not only feeds candida but also depletes the immune system, disturbs blood glucose levels, and prevents the absorption of nutrients that help control fungal growth. Irritable Bowel Syndrome is common in drinkers or those who have been heavy drinkers in the past. For some reason the obvious signs of fungal infections often do not appear until the person has cut down or stopped drinking. (It is not uncommon to see recovering alcoholics covered in fungal rashes. The rashes can be anywhere, but more commonly on the trunk and arms, and can persist for months.) It is obviously better for drinkers to abstain totally during candida treatment, however symptoms can improve if they limit their intake and pay more attention to their diet and general health, take antifungal substances, as well as nutritional supplements.

CHAPTER THREE

Allergies and Food Intolerance

An allergic reaction is an inflammatory response to a substance (an allergen) to which the body is exposed, either by inhalation, ingestion, or through contact with the skin. The allergen causes the body's own antibodies to assault the substance. This assault begins a chain reaction of chemical changes that causes swelling or irritation. The result is asthma, hives, hay fever, and eczema. Food allergies (such as peanuts) can cause more extreme reactions. Food allergens are caused by antibodies to food proteins and affect the immune system. They usually involve only one or two foods. Allergic symptoms can be severe enough sometimes to necessitate brief admission to the hospital. These include: itching; difficulty in breathing; swelling of the lips, tongue, and throat; and nausea. Allergic reactions to food are well-documented; what is less well documented is food intolerance.

Food Intolerance

Food intolerance, on the other hand, often occurs when foods that have been eaten regularly are stopped and cravings and other withdrawal symptoms develop. The diagnosis of food intolerance is not well recognized by traditional physicians, possibly because the symptoms can be vague and confused with other conditions, particularly psychological problems. (The patient is often dismissed as neurotic.) The symptoms of food intolerance look very much like those of candida overgrowth and the two conditions often co-exist. Symptoms include

- flushing, sweating after meals
- foul taste in the mouth, loss of taste
- sore mouth, mouth ulcers
- abnormal thirst
- asthma
- hives (nettle rash)
- inflamed digestive tract
- bloating
- continuous dull abdominal ache
- constipation
- diarrhea
- flattened stool
- feeling of never having a complete bowel movement
- itching anus
- frequency of urine
- urgency of stool
- feeling of the brain being swollen
- irritability, outburst of rage
- feeling "spaced out"
- anxiety or depression after eating certain foods
- chronic fatigue
- hyperactivity

Often these symptoms persist for years, with the sufferer either gaining weight from food cravings and fluid retention, or losing weight because of lack of appetite and anxiety over food. The cry is often, "All pleasure has gone from eating—just what can I eat?"

Children and Food Intolerance

Food intolerance in children is becoming increasingly common. Their immune systems cannot cope with modern living: pollution, poor diet, food additives, and too many antibiotics. They can also be affected by the health of the mother during pregnancy. Children with food intolerance can be pale and listless, or pale and hyperactive. Other symptoms are

- mental dullness
- black circles under the eyes
- recurrent ear, nose, and throat problems
- bedwetting
- sleep disturbances
- itchy nose
- excessive thirst
- vomiting
- constipation
- diarrhea
- hyperactivity
- aggression

Soy Products

Many adults cannot tolerate soy products so it is not surprising that it is high on the list of foods causing problems in children. Doctors often prescribe soy milk for babies intolerant to cow's milk. While some babies thrive on it, many don't. Both doctor and mother are often slow to suspect an intolerance to the substitute milk because the symptoms do not start immediately, and, in fact, after discontinuing the cow's milk there is often improvement for a time. However, soy milk seems an unnatural diet for infants when you consider that they take up to eight ounces at a feeding. Although high in nutrients, beans can be indigestible because they contain both starch and protein. Perhaps because of the amount of the milk consumed and the fact that they ingest it every day babies develop an intolerance to the soy milk, i.e., their immune system is constantly being bombarded by a foreign substance and does not have time to recover. The following is a good example of what has just been discussed.

> When Joseph was six months old I stopped breastfeeding and introduced cow's milk formula into his diet. He developed eczema that got progressively worse. After about eight weeks I decided to remove all cow's milk from his diet. As an alternative, my doctor recommended specially formulated baby soy milk available by prescription. The eczema improved considerably and I began using other soy products such as yogurt and custard. All went well, although I did notice Joseph now drank less milk (about half a pint daily). When he was 11 months Joseph caught a stomach bug and vomited and had diarrhea for several days. We gave him water only and he seemed to recover, although his bowel movements remained very loose with a very acrid, sour smell. After a week or so he vomited violently during the night but seemed fine the rest of the time.

> This continued for several weeks: violent vomiting during the night once or twice a week. Continued visits to the doctor were unhelpful; I was constantly told that babies were like that, or it was "just a bug."

> On his first birthday Joseph was very sick again, but this time he was listless, weak, and in a generally poor state for several days. His abdomen seemed swollen and around his anus was sore. I called the doctor and was told not to worry.

> After a few days on water only Joseph recovered but by now we were anxious; he seemed to be getting thinner and each ill-

ness seemed to last longer and would be more severe than the last. This pattern continued through December and into January. The bouts of sickness got worse and more frequent and Joseph got weaker. In between attacks I was giving him as much soy milk as possible in a vain effort to "build him up." Finally, in January, he was so ill that I demanded hospital admission. This time his abdomen and feet were very swollen. He was there for five days and had blood and stool tests. The doctors found nothing and were baffled by Joseph's condition, which by now had improved, although his tummy was still swollen and his rectum remained very red and sore.

I didn't know whether to feel relieved or not. Joseph was discharged and I was told to give him plenty of soy milk and to come back if he became ill again.

By now I was determined to get to the root of the problem and was convinced that: (a) The original stomach bug back in October had for some reason upset Joseph's system so much that he was now unable to tolerate or digest something, but what? Something that had been okay before he got the bug? (b) The solution lay in the elimination of something and the sorting out of Joseph's system.

I was continually searching for answers and by now was so stressed myself I didn't know what to do. It was at this point I decided to seek help from "alternative" practitioners. I took Joseph to see a homeopathic doctor and also consulted a nutrition counselor. Both told me to stop the soy milk and replace it with goat milk. I diluted the goat milk at first and built it up to full strength over a week. Within 24 hours we noticed an incredible difference in Joseph. Soy milk had been the culprit all those months. Joseph seemed almost relieved that we had finally solved the problem. He was altogether happier; his skin cleared; his bowel movements were normal; and with the help of homeopathic remedies and a careful diet (wheat and yeast-free) he returned to normal. The counselor asked if Joseph had ever had oral thrush. He had it three times during *the early weeks of his life, and I also have a problem with candida.*

It is now six months since Joseph was ill. He is thriving, his weight is back to normal, and he is a really happy child. His eczema has cleared and he now tolerates cow's milk products. When I look back at the whole experience I think that the worst part of it was that not one of the doctors I saw, even at the hospital, suspected intolerance to soy milk. I have since heard of several similar cases. Why is the medical profession unaware of this problem?

Luke's Story

Luke was breastfed until he was five months old and was a contented, cheerful baby. While he was being weaned he became fretful, wheezy, and had skin rashes. His mother figured this was from teething. By the time he was two years old he was hyperactive and slept fitfully. His mother thought this was the terrible twos and did not seek help until he started nursery school. The teacher said he was aggressive and difficult to control. When his mother consulted the doctor she was advised to keep him on an additive-free diet. This helped but she still felt that his behavior was not normal. He could not settle down to play with toys or listen to stories the way her two older children had done. Although she had no doubt that he was intelligent, she noted that at times he was vague, far away, and in her words "difficult to reach." He was referred to an allergy unit and was found to be intolerant to sugar and anything in the onion family.

One day he came home from having a snack with a friend and appeared "in a world of his own." He climbed on the kitchen table and leapt back and forth to the sink. This was something he had never done before. He became aggressive when he was restrained. His mother learned later that he had eaten a vegetable burger containing leeks. There had been other similar episodes after birthday parties. An exclusion diet greatly improved his symptoms, he was calmer, could concentrate, and was now quite happy to play alone with his toys. He progressed well and only lapsed when he strayed from his diet.

Contributing Factors in Food Intolerance in Children

- Genetic influence
- Stressed immune system
- Environmental factors
- Harmful bacteria, candida overgrowth, parasites in the gut
- Drugs
- Inflammation in the gut
- Damage to the gut wall—leaky gut
- Lack of hydrochloric acid or enzymes
- Disturbance of pancreatic function
- Low levels to butyric acid made in the gut

Food Intolerance—the Candida Connection

Some practitioners believe that overgrowth of candida in the bowel is the major cause of food intolerance. Others believe it is the other way around, i.e, stress and environmental factors cause food intolerance and then candida takes over when the immune system is too weak to fight back. These practitioners treat the food intolerance first, believing the immune system recovers enough to cope with the candida. They identify the offending substances using muscle testing (kinesiology), and then stimulate the body's own defense mechanism by giving homeopathic doses of the allergens. This is known as desensitization. For a practitioner who uses this approach in your area see "Useful Addresses" at the end of the book.

Food Allergy Testing

During the past several years the availability and range of tests for food intolerance has increased. Formerly tests were mainly available for asthma and hayfever sufferers who were inhaling allergens. Following are some of the tests now available:

THE SKIN PRICK

This is the standard test to determine the reaction to common allergens. A drop of the allergen is placed on the skin, which is then pricked or scratched. If the patient is sensitive to the allergen there is a swelling of the area, known as the wheal-and-flare response. This works well for inhaled allergens such as pollens and dust but is unreliable for food intolerance.

INTRADERMAL INJECTIONS

These go deeper into the skin than the prick and are more reliable. If the body does not react to the substance it produces a small wheal that soon disappears. A positive reaction increases in size and becomes white and hard.

NEUTRALIZATION

This treatment is based on finding a dilution of the offending substance that will "turn off" the allergic reaction by its influence on the immune system. The reason this works is unknown, but it closely parallels the homeopathic principle of like curing like, that is, the correct dilution of the allergen effects a cure.

ENZYME-POTENTIATED DESENSITIZATION (EPD)

Enzyme Potentiated Desensitization is a method of treatment using extremely small doses of allergens to desensitize people from their allergies. This test is more likely to be used by doctors who work in the area of clinical nutrition. It has been effective for food, inhalant, and chemical sensitivities. One advantage of this method is that it is only needed about once every three months, and less and less as the immune system recovers. Contact the American EPD Society (see "Useful Addresses") for more information.

Butyric Acid for Food Intolerance

In a healthy gut adequate amounts of butyric acid (also known as butanoic acid) are made by the action of bacteria on dietary fiber (fermentation). (This fatty acid also appears in large amounts in breast milk.) The lining of the bowel has some of the fastest growing cells in the body and butyrates have been shown to supply their energy needs and promote natural healing. Low levels of production of butyric acid could precipitate bowel disease in susceptible persons. Butyric Acid Complex is available in capsule form. It should not be used by persons suffering from gastric ulcers or gastritis (inflammation of the stomach). Patients who have been taking from two to four capsules of butyrates at every meal have experienced freedom from many food sensitivities after a period of seven to fourteen days.

Will the Doctor Be Able to Help?

The medical evidence for food sensitivities remains controversial mainly because there has been a lack of properly controlled studies; the evidence is mainly anecdotal. Some people have consulted their doctors for years and have only been given prescriptions for antacids, preparations for constipation, diarrhea, or colic while routine checkups in hospitals fail to discover the cause of their distress. Some have been referred by their doctors to allergists and have found this helpful in determining which are the offending foods. Others have found the tests for food allergies unreliable (particularly skin pricks) and have found more success following exclusion diets and their own intuition. (CAUTION: Long periods on very restricted diets can lead to vitamin and mineral deficiencies.)

If you can afford to see a doctor who specializes in clinical nutrition you will find that the blood or muscle testing you are given pinpoint your allergies more accurately, and you are likely to be given reasonable guidance on diet and supplements. If you have to rely on your own efforts, do not be disappointed; many people have been in the same position and have done very well.

How Can I Find Out Which Food Is Upsetting Me?

The only reliable way to find out which are the offending substances is to abstain from foods that you normally eat every day, particularly the ones that make you feel ill after eating, and see what happens to your symptoms.

The Pulse Test

You could also try the pulse test. A rise in the pulse can denote food intolerance. Before using the pulse test, avoid the suspected food for at least five days (some practitioners recommend a month), then take your resting pulse before having a generous helping of the food. Place your palm upward and press the outer aspect of the wrist with your forefinger, in line with the thumb, and you will feel your pulse. Count the number of beats in 15 seconds then multiply by four. This will give the number of beats per minute. If it is raised ten or more beats ten minutes after you have eaten a certain food keep a record of this in a food diary. Take it again after about an hour. Don't rely on memory: keep a record each day of your meals, snacks, and drinks, and note any symptoms. Some people don't need to wait ten minutes to take their pulse before their familiar allergic symptoms—heartbeat skipping, headache, wheezing, stuffy nose and so on—descend on them. For some people it only takes two to three minutes. In general the abdominal symptoms (bloating and discomfort) take longer to manifest themselves.

Some doctors say the pulse test is unreliable because people may get anxious thinking the food is going to upset them, creating a rise in their pulse rate. However, this does not explain why patients in blind tests have reactions when they are unaware of what foods they are being given.

If the Challenge Is Too Uncomfortable

There are products on the market that provide symptomatic relief of food intolerance. You might find one in your health food store. You can try one teaspoonful of sodium bicarbonate alone in a glass of warm water if this is your only option.

Some people find that eating a large helping of a food they know they can tolerate somehow neutralizes the negative effect of a food they are intolerant to.

Keeping Cool

Reactions to food intolerance are worse when you are hot. To cool down, try splashing your face with cold water, having a cool shower or bath, or resting with an ice pack on your head or abdomen (don't shudder—this can be surprisingly comforting). A good alternative to an ice pack is an unopened bag of frozen peas. (*Note:* The peas cannot be returned to the freezer for consumption but can be used again as an ice pack.) To prevent ice burn, packs should be wrapped in a thin cloth such as a cloth napkin or tea towel.

Food Rotation Diet

The principle of this diet is rotation and diversification of food. It is based on the fact that you are most likely to become intolerant to foods you have eaten all your life. Food rotation allows your immune system to recover by not bombarding it with the same allergens every day. Some people react to so many foods they can't possibly exclude them all from their diet so they eat most foods, but only once every four days. The body seems to be able to cope with this method and many people do well using this diet. It is, of course, tedious, as all diets are. There are many books available that describe food intolerance in detail (see "Further Reading" at the end of this book for some suggestions).

Obesity, Candida, and Food Intolerance

There are several factors that could lead to obesity in candida suffers, including altered hormone levels due to the candida, as well as a genetic inability to cope with grains. But sugar and bread craving—the candida constantly "crying out" for its favorite food—is probably the main cause of obesity in candida sufferers. Many overweight sufferers do not make significant progress until they remove all grains from their diet for at least four weeks. No matter how carefully they have dieted, even on one slice of bread a day, they cannot lose weight. Weight loss is often dramatic when they go grain-free (with the possible exception of brown rice and rice cakes). Fluid retention disappears and bloated abdomens improve, even if their caloric intake remains the same.

When you eat foods your body is intolerant to, the cells react by protecting themselves with extra fluid. This excess fluid can dramatically increase your weight. In addition, the addiction/allergy connection is closely related; you may crave the very foods that are causing your weight problem.

Some people find it difficult to lose weight because they do not eat enough protein to boost their metabolism and keep their blood sugar levels stable. This also makes them lethargic, compounding their ability to exercise. Vegetarians are often in this group. Overweight people often have low essential vitamin and mineral intake and have a toxic colon problem as well.

Being Underweight and Having Candida

If you are underweight, and particularly if your appetite is poor, consult your doctor or a nutritionist before embarking on an anti-candida diet. If your appetite is good and you can eat much larger helpings of the allowed foods, and if weight loss does not continue (you could expect some at first), you could see how you fare. Underweight people would do well to investigate the desensitization approach (page 26) that only calls for a reduction in sugar and salt.

Chemical Intolerance

Substances that cause the gut to swell and give rise to other symptoms of intolerance don't always gain access to the body through the mouth, but are inhaled or absorbed through the skin. You should become more aware of the chemicals you spray on your head, under your arms, up your nose, and on your skin. It is best to use simple non-perfumed toiletries and not buy aerosol cans. Antiperspirants stop natural detoxification through the skin so use a simple deodorant. Most essential oils are antiseptic, and tea tree (see pages 59–60) is available as a deodorant stick. Some oils come in a carrier oil, such as jojoba, and can be used as a perfume. They smell wonderful and you are much less likely to be intolerant to them.

There is a range of ecological cleaning products available that are better for the chemically intolerant—as well as safer for the environment. If you suffer from chemical intolerance throw out your household cleaning agents and buy simple soaps (nonbiological detergents) and old-fashioned wax furniture polish instead of spray cans. If you cannot find a safe product make sure you immerse the nozzle of your container under water so that you don't inhale the droplets. Research has confirmed that traces of dish detergent can irritate the bowel lining so it is important to rinse your dishes very carefully. It is very common for people with chemical allergies to get a tight chest while washing the dishes. Avoid garden chemicals as much as possible. Frequent hoeing is safer than using noxious weed killers and dish detergent liquid is quite effective for ridding your plants of aphids (unfortunately, some plants do not like ecological products). If you have to paint or use wood preservatives, make sure your working space is well ventilated and that you take frequent breaks. (See "Further Reading" on page 188 for books on natural cleaning substances and natural gardening.)

Environmental Hazards

Today the world abounds in potential allergens. Inhalation of brake fluid on trains causes swollen eyes, headaches, and abdominal symptoms in some chemically allergic people. Traveling by car can also be a problem. (Keep the windows closed and if possible buy a car ionizer [see page 78]; they are inexpensive and well worth the effort. Make frequent stops to escape fumes.)

Chemical inhalants from plastics, adhesives, and flooring in shopping areas can cause symptoms in some people. Printer's ink, tobacco smoke, gas, oil, factory fumes, formaldehyde (air fresheners), particleboard furniture, synthetic carpets—although the fumes from these do decrease with time—are also implicated. In addition to manmade allergens, allergens in nature such as pollens and dust mites can cause problems.

A Toxic Colon

A toxic colon is a major factor in the development of food intolerance leading to chronic ill health. You cannot expect to be well if the main organ responsible for ridding the body of toxic waste is underfunctioning. When the colon is irritated by diet, stress, drugs, chemicals, and other substances, it tries to protect itself by producing more mucus. This additional mucus can bind with the sludge from refined foods, such as white flour, and build up on the wall of the bowel, narrowing the lumen. This layer of gluey, hardened feces can weigh several pounds and is a good place for harmful organisms to breed. Do not think because you have regular bowel movements or even diarrhea that you have escaped this problem. The stool can pass daily through a dirty colon and leave the accumulated residue on the walls behind. There is no need to get panicky about the amount of weighty garbage you might be carrying around with you: there is a great deal you can do about it.

How This Toxic Layer Can Affect the Body

The local effects of this poisonous residue are irritation and inflammation of the colon: the general reactions include diarrhea, constipation, fatigue, headaches, dull eyes, poor skin, spots, aching muscles, joint pains, and depression. The poisons circulate via the blood through the lymphatic system to all parts of the body. (Healthy lymphatic fluid serves to nourish cells not fed by blood vessels and kills off harmful organisms, carrying away the refuse.) If the body has to pump excessive toxic waste around for any length of time then it is not surprising that it sometimes gives up, allowing the disease process to take over.

When the muscles of the colon wall lose tone, ballooning, or the formation of pouches called diverticula, result, leading to a condition known as diverticulosis. The food trapped in these pockets creates a breeding ground for bacteria. The result can be diverticulitis, an infection where there is often a fever and acute abdominal pain. This condition needs medical help.

Cleansing the Colon

Colon cleansing is the first step on the road to recovery. When you have cleansed your colon and restored the balance of the good and bad bacteria, when you have adequate production of enzymes, and your dietary intake and internal production of vitamins is correct, your food intolerance should greatly improve or disappear. I believe the benefits of colon cleansing are many, not only in terms of health, but also as it relates to appearance: the skin looks vibrant; cellulite, water retention, and blemishes disappear; and the whites of the eyes regain a youthful clearness. How quickly you want to clean out your colon is your choice. Some people are so tired of being under par they are willing to endure the effects of rapid cleansing. Possible side effects from this procedure include migraine headaches, blinding headaches, nausea, or flu, aches and pains, fever, exhaustion, and nervous symptoms such as anxiety, panic attacks, irritability, weepiness, and even profound depression. The worst of this would be over in approximately five days.

You might prefer a more gradual process: changing to a clean diet over a period of several weeks. Start with a diet of 50 percent raw food along with a teaspoonful of linseed (available from health food stores) or two level teaspoonsful of Metamucil or Citrucel, bulking agents available at pharmacies or grocery stores. You can chew the linseed to release the nutrients. Metamucil or Citrucel is easier to swallow if you mix it with yogurt. Water is an essential element in the cleansing process; aim for two quarts per day while you are cleansing the colon, unless this conflicts with advice from your doctor. Start off the day with at least a half pint of water, preferably hot, before breakfast. Many people are afraid to consume that much water because they retain fluid, but some practitioners believe that the body retains fluid when it does not get enough; it tries to hang on to its ration.

How Long Does It Take to Clean the Colon?

It is unlikely that you will have a cleansed colon within a couple of weeks: it could take months. You will know when things are happening: your skin and eyes will look clearer, your digestion will improve, you will have more energy, and nagging aches and pains that have been around for years will disappear. You could feel mentally better too, clear-headed, and less jumpy.

This process is described in my book *Irritable Bowel Syndrome & Diverticulosis* (Thorsons, 1992). *New Again!* by Anna Selby (Ulysses Press, 1999) offers a 28-day detoxification plan that includes a juice fast and healthy regimen for getting your body back on track. If you also want to lose weight with clean eating using a common-sense approach read *Fit For Life* by Harvey and Marilyn Diamond.

COLONIC IRRIGATION

Most people think of colon irrigation as a nightmarish experience. It is far from this. In fact, it is a very quick and efficient way to loosen impacted feces and wash away toxins. It also obviates many of the unpleasant symptoms of detoxification. Here's what happens: a sterile tube is inserted into the rectum and filtered water washes around the colon. An evacuation tube removes the water, taking with it years of accumulated debris and mucus.

If you want to find a practitioner in your area, contact the International Association for Colon Hydrotherapy (see "Useful Addresses").

CAN VITAMINS HELP?

An adequate intake of B vitamins is essential for a healthy immune system. Niacin (vitamin B_3) is particularly helpful. Niacin helps the detoxification process by stimulating circulation. It often produces a harmless flushing or prickling of the skin, which disappears in less than an hour of consumption. (Nicotinamide is a form of B_3 that does not cause flushing.) Niacin has been shown not only to prevent the development of allergies, but it also helps alleviate cramps and sugar or alcohol craving. It has also been found to help nervous symptoms because it closely resembles the group of drugs called the benzodiazepines (Valium, Ativan, etc.). (Note: Niacin supplements should be taken carefully; amounts over 500 milligrams daily may cause liver damage.)

The B vitamins are synergistic: they depend on each other for absorption (vitamin B_3 needs vitamin B_6). You should not take any of them in isolation without professional guidance. It is also vital that you choose yeast-free preparations. Some people with bowel problems find even the purest non-allergenic brands give them problems. If this happens to you, cut down the recommended dose and build up gradually, or take them two to three times weekly. (See pages 68–70 for more information about supplements.)

CHAPTER FOUR

Other Fungal Conditions

Cystitis

It is thought that candida is able to invade the bladder wall in the same manner that it attacks the lining of the bowel or the vagina. I have seen hundreds of people whose symptoms have failed to respond to antibiotics and whose urine analysis proved negative. Their symptoms finally did, however, respond to antifungal medication or to self-help anti-candida methods.

Fungal Cystitis

People with fungal cystitis have different symptoms than the "ordinary" cystitis (bacterial) sufferer. Bacterial cystitis episodes are usually isolated attacks, causing pain or burning during urination. Urine from a bacterial infection usually has an unpleasant smell and often contains pus or blood. Urgency and frequency are also features of bacterial cystitis. This symptom picture usually responds quite quickly to antibiotics. By contrast, fungal cystitis does not. In fungal cystitis the symptoms tend to be less dramatic. There is discomfort in the bladder and the urethra that is made worse by drinking citrus juices, alcohol, strong coffee, some soft drinks, and also by yeasty, sugary foods as well as some vitamin supplements, particularly vitamins C and B complex. It is true that a bladder inflamed by bacteria or a virus would also react to acidic drinks, but it is unlikely that normal cystitis sufferers would be affected by eating bread or other foods normally included in their diet.

Fungal cystitis might be the only symptom of candida, although it is more commonly seen in people who have fungal infections in other sites such as the gut, vagina, or nail beds. (An irritated bladder can also be a feature of food intolerance.)

An important point to remember is that urine specimens sent for an analysis are not generally tested for fungus without a special request. If you identify your symptoms with those of fungal cystitis it would be wise to ask your doctor if a fungal test could be included in the test.

Proprietary Medicines for Cystitis

These can bring temporary relief to an inflamed bladder but should not be used for long periods of time. They work by making the urine alkaline and ease the inflammation in much the same way an antacid soothes an irritated gastric lining. As with antacids, it is unwise to use these preparations for prolonged periods because they upset the delicate acid-alkaline balance of the body and can lead to further problems. In the case of fungal cystitis, these medications may make you feel more comfortable but since candida thrives in an alkaline medium it could eventually compound your problem. Some preparations contain citric acid.

Natural Remedies for Cystitis

Women are more prone to cystitis than men because they have a shorter urethra (tube leading from the bladder), allowing harmful organisms from the bowel to ascend into the bladder. In the article "Urinary Tract Infection and the Potential for a Natural Prophylactic Treatment," the author notes the effect of cranberry juice on urinary tract infections. The article asserts that it can help prevent infections by preventing harmful bacteria, particularly E. coli, from attaching to the lining of the bladder:

> There seems to be little doubt that cranberry juice can be extremely valuable in the prophylaxis [prevention] of urinary tract infections, especially for patients with recurrence. It is probable that the relief of acute infection will always lie in the domain of antibiotics, but as well as other side effects, they do diminish the host's own defenses against the recurrence of the disease. Overall, urinary tract infection is such a major problem, notably of female health, that any effective addition to the armory of the practitioner would be very welcome. One advantage of cranberry juice is that it cannot possibly do any harm—only good.

Cranberry juice is very popular as a remedy for bladder problems. However, it is important to get a brand that does not have sugar added. These brands can be found in health food stores and some specialty markets.

Homeopathy, herbs, and essential oils are also used for the relief of cystitis.

Drink as much water (preferably bottled) as you can and take warm baths at the slightest sign of discomfort in the bladder or urethra. Sometimes a hot-water bottle on the lower back or abdomen helps.

The bladder can become irritated by eating or drinking something you are intolerant to even if there is no bacterial or fungal infection.

For more on the management of cystitis see "Further Reading" at the back of this book.

Candida and ME (Myalgic Encephalomyelitis)

ME is a chronic illness thought to be viral in origin that depresses the immune system. This suppression allows other opportunist viruses, bacteria, or fungi to step in and produce a bewildering, debilitating illness. The central nervous system can also be affected, causing transient paralysis, speech and eating problems, as well as a loss of balance. ME is characterized by bouts of extreme tiredness in the muscles and brain that are not alleviated by rest. It can start with an illness like glandular fever or flu. This understandably gives rise to feelings of hopelessness and depression. Sometimes it is so severe people have to give up work for a time.

Sufferers have often been classified as malingerers or hypochondriacs and many have been very harshly treated by their medical practitioners. ME is often mistaken for "nerves" because the symptoms include anxiety, depression, and lethargy.

Research on this condition has provided few answers in the area of conventional medicine, except where nutritional therapy has been combined with antidepressant medication, particularly the drug amitriptyline. Overall, however, the best results have been reported with the approach used by clinical nutritionists who treat nutritional deficiencies (ME sufferers are often found to be low in magnesium), candida, and food intolerance.

Treatment

Because the immune system is suppressed in ME sufferers, yeast-related problems and allergies are very common. Full recovery cannot take place without these conditions being treated.

Other important aspects of treatment are rest, a healthy diet, nutritional supplements (during severe illness or times of stress the body demands an increase in essential minerals and vitamins), fresh air, daylight, and keeping the bowel as clean as possible by preventing constipation and restoring the normal balance of bacteria to the gut. Any therapy that promotes relaxation and natural healing is also recommended. Tranquilizers rarely help in the treatment of ME; they merely add more poisons to a body that is already struggling to excrete the poisons caused by the virus. However, sometimes a nighttime dose of a sedative antidepressant is helpful when insomnia is severe and where normal sleep-wake cycles are trying to be established.

Sufferers need to be believed, reassured that they will recover in time, and to have the nature of the illness fully explained to them. Check the internet for up-to-date information on this condition. For further information about ME see "Useful Addresses" and "Further Reading" at the back of the book.

Fungal Skin Problems

The most important point to remember about skin problems is that they generally start on the *inside* of the body. Localized infections are a sign that the immune system is not as healthy as it could be. No matter how many times skin problems clear up with creams and ointments they will recur if the body's defenses are not kept in good working order.

Candida is not responsible for all fungal skin problems; more than one parasitic yeast may invade the body when the immune system is low. For example, nail bed and scalp ringworm are due to dermatophyte fungi (tinea). While they are often seen in people with chronic candida they require a different systemic and topical treatment. Be sure to see your doctor if you have candida-like symptoms, or skin or nail-bed infections that do not clear up with anti-candida measures.

Some skin problems can be distressing, particularly if they are on the face. They usually take the form of a scaly red rash at the sides of the nose and between the eyebrows. If the rash is severe it can extend across the cheeks and can have the appearance of sunburn. The hands can also become very dry. Very often skin flare-ups are associated with stress and it is difficult to say how much is fungal in origin and how much can be attributed to the candida in the gut that results in vitamin deficiencies. It is probably both. Not only does the immune system have to work harder during stressful times to keep the candida under control but there is also a need for an increased intake of some vitamins, particularly the B vitamins. This is why combining antifungal treatment with vitamins is more effective than either treatment alone.

Athlete's Foot

This infection is characterized by itching and redness between the toes. The skin can be flaked, cracked, or moist. Footbaths with tea tree oil, the application of neat tea tree oil, or creams plus strict foot hygiene are effective (see page 47).

Nail Bed Infections

These infections can be very stubborn and take several months to clear. Topical application alone is not usually enough. Internal treatment plus regular application of neat tea tree oil or an antifungal cream (not Nystatin) is necessary (see page 47).

Acne

This disfiguring condition is caused by a hormonal influence affecting the sebaceous glands. It produces blackheads and pustules on the face, neck, and shoulders. Acne occurs mainly during adolescence but can occur later in life when drugs alter hormone levels. It is thought that overproduction of hormones encourages fungal growth and it has been noticed that people having treatment for candidiasis often lose all trace of acne. Persons who have had long-term antibiotic treatment for acne in their youth often suffer severe candida problems later on. Acne sufferers are also often found to be zinc deficient; niacinamide is a major nutrient involved in the repair of the skin because it opens the vascular system, which supplies the skin with nutrients.

Psoriasis

This is a distressing chronic skin condition characterized by raised, red, scaly lesions. Some scientists believe that it is genetic in origin; others favor hormonal influences, raised cholesterol levels, allergic reactions to food or drugs; others see stress as the major factor, with the condition often appearing up to two years after a traumatic event. Medical science admits that existing treatments are inadequate and that some of the drugs used have adverse effects. Nutritional therapists have long associated this condition with a depressed immune system and/or candida. Sufferers are often found to have a marked zinc deficiency.

Some doctors have seen the candida/psoriasis connection for some time. Professor E. William Rosenburg, dermatologist of the University of Tennessee College of Medicine in Memphis, claims a 75 percent success rate within four months on antifungal drugs and sugar/refined carbohydrate/yeast-free diet. Nutritionists recommend a diet high in raw vegetables, fruit, and oily fish such as herring and mackerel. One study attributed the low level of psoriasis among Eskimos to high levels of omega fatty acids found in their diet. Herbal remedies and homeopathy can also be helpful in treating this condition.

CHAPTER FIVE

Case Histories

In this chapter I will highlight what could be considered minor problems, in a medical sense, but problems that still cause a great deal of distress and impair the quality of life. The persistent nature of some of these problems, and their tendency to recur year after year, can lead sufferers to a feeling of hopelessness and helplessness.

Swollen Sore Genitals

When a 22-year-old male student came for help he described his life as completely miserable; his penis was so swollen and sore that walking and sitting through lectures was awkward. When he was in his room he only wore a long T-shirt, outdoors a loose tracksuit; it was impossible for him to wear jeans, his normal attire. He was also anxious, frustrated, and depressed. He had no social life and was very worried about the future.

He had been seeing his doctor for several months and had initially been given antibiotics, followed by a course of antifungal drugs and cortisone cream. The antifungal treatment helped but within a few days of stopping treatment the symptoms returned. He was finally sent to a clinic for Sexually Transmitted Disease where he was told he had both bacterial and fungal infections. He was given a course of antibiotics and antifungal medication, which were more effective than the antifungal treatment alone. Again, once treatment stopped the symptoms returned.

He finally contacted a candida counselor who asked about his diet and food cravings. It was then that he realized how much he craved cheese and marmite sandwiches and a daily pint of beer. He ate the sandwiches, which were the mainstay of his diet, because they were convenient and economical. On reflection he realized that hunger was not the only reason he craved his sandwiches because he also ate a sandwich after dining out—he realized it was the candida scream-ing for its favorite "food."

The counselor offered several suggestions. After reviewing the options he chose the garlic method (see page 50) and made a half-hearted attempt at the candida diet. Two weeks after starting the treatment his condition had improved some, but he felt he would have to be stricter about his diet. He ended up taking acidophilus and yeast-free mineral and vitamin supplements. Four weeks later he called to say he was doing very well, except when he reverted to his old habits.

Abdominal Symptoms Plus Recurrent Ear Infections

A 39-year-old female had successfully withdrawn from tranquilizers after taking them for ten years. Three months after withdrawal she complained of a bloated abdomen, a constant feeling of imminent cys-titis, and an ear infection. The ear discharged a watery fluid which dried into a crystalline deposit on her skin that reached nearly to her chin. The skin became inflamed and had the appearance of a burn.

She was prescribed three different courses of antibiotics without any benefit before a swab was sent to the laboratory. The result confirmed she had a fungal infection. She was given antifungal ear drops and cream for her skin. The ear symptoms needed prolonged treatment but eventually cleared up. Her abdominal symptoms and urinary symptoms persisted until she went on the anti-candida diet.

Skin Problems: Pityriasis Rosea

Elizabeth had a history of being given antibiotics for ear infections as a child, and as an adult for a kidney infection. For several years after the kidney infection she had feelings of impending cystitis, often associated with stress or eating certain foods.

After a particularly stressful period in her life she noticed a slight dry rash. It worsened over a period of ten days until it separated into round red patches about the size of nickels. The patches looked like cigarette burns and appeared only on the trunk of her body. Itching was a problem, especially when she was hot.

The doctor diagnosed pityriasis rosea. She said it was caused by an airborne virus, possibly picked up on a bus, and there was no cure. She was told it would clear up on its own accord within about three months. Elizabeth was horrified at the thought of having such a disfiguring, uncomfortable rash for so long. She also realized it would prevent her from swimming or doing any exercise that would make her hot.

Elizabeth remembered that her cousin had been diagnosed with the same condition, but her doctor had attributed it to a fungal infection. She bought a book on candida and started on the anti-candida diet immediately. She was very strict about sugar (even fruit), bread, and cheese; she was not quite as strict with wine and diet Coke. Vegetables, fish, lamb, and free-range corn-fed eggs were the mainstay of her diet. Other red meats and eggs were avoided because antibiotics are included in their feed.

To alleviate the itching she used essential oils of lavender and tea tree, three drops of each, in a daily bath and she applied two drops of each oil mixed with one teaspoon of olive oil twice daily to the rash. She also went to a tanning salon every three or four days.

After a telephone counseling session with a nutritionist Elizabeth started taking supplements a few days later, including caprylic acid, superdophillus, as well as herbal tablets. Psyllium husks were recommended as part of a bowel cleansing program and she also drank the antifungal herbal tea pau d'Arco. Pau d'Arco is a biochemically complex antifungal tea containing lapachol made from the unsprayed bark (the tree is unharmed by the harvest) of the Inca Bow Tree. It is also known as taheebo and lapacho. The Inca Indians made bows from these trees and drank the tea from the bark. During the first week the rash actually got worse, but after ten days there was a slight improvement, with definite progress a few days later. The rash was most stubborn around the armpits and stomach, where her body was warmest. Elizabeth soon could see the rash clearing before her eyes, seemingly retreating inward. Her story illustrates how attacking fungal skin infections from both the inside and out can achieve rapid results.

Severe Itching of the Scrotum and Groin

John had an unbearably itchy rash around his anus, scrotum, and up into his groin. He was losing sleep, becoming irritable, and finding it impossible to sit still. His work was suffering because of poor concentration. Sitting in cold water was the only way he could ease the itching. The creams he had been prescribed worked to some extent, but the benefits did not last.

He was questioned about his diet and lifestyle; both seemed healthy. He ate plenty of vegetables, salads, fruit, and fish, got adequate exercise, and was a non-smoker who drank moderately on weekends. However, the source of the problem was revealed when he was asked about stress at work. Things had been a bit hectic at work since Christmas so on a colleague's recommendation he took brewer's yeast tablets for additional B vitamins. When asked if he had associated the onset of his symptoms with the taking of the tablets he realized it had not occurred to him. He thought brewer's yeast was an old-fashioned, healthy addition to his diet and could do no harm.

On reflection he saw the connection. All he did to cure himself was to stop taking the brewer's yeast and drink lots of water. Within two days later he was much improved; a week later his skin was back to normal.

It can be seen from John's story that fungal problems can arise in people who are perfectly healthy. Something as simple as a dietary change can cause the candida in the bowel to multiply out of control.

Chemical Intolerance

Adrian, who had been diagnosed with ME (Myalgic Encephalomyelitis), had been unable to work for three months. He started having bowel problems while traveling in India. After being home a year, the bowel problems had lessened but he seemed to be allergic to everything in sight. Paint, cigarette smoke, or even working in the garden shed or in the garden on a damp day could make him feel weak and exhausted for several days. He began to feel like a prisoner; his wife said he was neurotic; his self-esteem was at an all-time low.

Information from an ME self-help group gave him hope. He then saw a clinical nutritionist and after six months of antifungal nutritional therapy he felt back to his former self.

CHAPTER SIX

Looking for Answers

Antifungal Drugs

Antifungal drugs are effective but some do not come without their own set of problems.

- *Diflucan* (fluconazole) is increasingly being used for candida. *Be sure to check with your pharmacist for possible interactions if you are taking other drugs.* Also ask about other contraindications. (People often consult nutritionists for antifungal substances after being treated with this drug. This is not only because of the toxic reactions, but because of a rapid return of the candida as soon as the drug is discontinued.)

- *Amphotericin* (fungizone) is used for systemic fungal infections and is effective against most fungi and yeasts. It is, however, toxic and side effects are common. They include digestive upsets, headaches, and joint pains.

- *Grifulvin* is well absorbed in the gut and is often used when infections of the skin, scalp, and nails have failed to respond to creams and lotions. The side effects include headaches, digestive upsets, and sensitivity to light.

- The imidozole group—clotrimazole, econazole, ketonconzole (Nizoral), and miconazole—are active against a wide range of fungi and yeasts. Oral use, except for miconazole, is usually restricted to severe resistant infections. The drugs in this group are used widely in pessary, cream, spray, and powder forms. Many are available over the counter in pharmacies. They include *Lotrimin* (clotrimazole) and *Monistat* (miconazole).

- *Nystatin* (sold under the brand names Mycolog, Mycostatin, Mytrex, Nilstat, and Nystex), an older drug, is used for intestinal, vaginal, and skin infections due to candida. The side effects are fewer than those of other antifungal drugs. However, the Herxheimer reaction, or dieback, can occur. (As the drug kills the yeast cells they burst and release toxins into the bloodstream. If this is done too rapidly the effect can be similar to the flu: raised temperature, headaches, nausea, aches, and pains.) The problem can be minimized by gradually building up to the recommended dose or by reducing the amount of candida in the bowel by careful dieting for about a month before drug treatment. Some tablets do not dissolve until they reach the large intestine, missing infection elsewhere in the digestive tract. This could be helped by crushing the tablets and putting them in water. When Nystatin powder is used it is much easier to graduate the dose and it also treats the entire digestive tract.

One of the problems with these drugs is that they can lead to the development of stronger strains of candida that are drug-resistant. A vicious circle begins: higher doses are needed, which then weaken the immune system.

Prescribed Drugs that Favor the Growth of Candida

ANTIBIOTICS

Why antibiotics encourage candida overgrowth is easily understood. As has been said before, antibiotics are not selective: they destroy both useful and harmful bacteria simultaneously.

THE CONTRACEPTIVE PILL

There are two explanations as to why contraceptive pills might encourage candida: disturbances in hormone levels and abnormal glucose (sugar) tolerance. In women who take the pill the prevalence of abnormal glucose (sugar) tolerance is increased from approximately 4 to 35 percent. As in diabetes, if the blood glucose levels are raised (hyperglycemia) there is more "food" for the candida.

CORTICOSTEROIDS

Taking corticosteroids disturbs the hormone level. In addition, these drugs have a much greater influence than other groups of drugs upon glucose tolerance. Drugs such as Prednisone, steroid asthma inhalers, and even creams in large doses can have this same effect. This increase in hormone level can lead to overgrowth of candida in the body.

OTHER DRUGS THAT EFFECT GLUCOSE LEVELS AND PROMOTE CANDIDA

These include diuretics, beta blockers, cimetidine (Tagamet), and ranitidine (Zantac). (Cimetidine and ranitidine are extremely useful for the treatment of gastric ulcers and have saved countless people from surgery. Unfortunately, because they are considered safe, they have been abused in general practice. They are often prescribed for the slightest sign of gastric disturbance, without a thought being given to the patient's eating habits or lifestyle, and repeat prescriptions are issued for years without reassessment of the patient's condition.)

LAXATIVES

Overuse of strong laxatives prevents the absorption of essential nutrients and alters the natural bowel flora. The anecdotal evidence suggesting that these drugs can cause candidiasis is overwhelming.

Tranquilizers, Irritable Bowel Syndrome, and Chronic Candidiasis

To the writer's knowledge, there have been no medical studies done on the adverse effects of the gastrointestinal system from medium- or long-term use of tranquilizers, but anecdotal evidence reporting gastrointestinal problems from tranquilizer self-help groups cannot be ignored, and no doubt in time there will be scientific research to confirm such findings.

What tranquilizers and sleeping pills do to the gut is unclear, but there is no doubt in my mind that a high percentage of users develop Irritable Bowel Syndrome and systemic candidiasis, or some manifestation of fungal infections, either during therapy or during withdrawal. The symptoms can persist for many years after complete withdrawal of the drugs. More gastrointestinal problems have been reported in people taking lorazepam (Ativan) than the other drugs in the group such as diazepam (Valium). It has been shown that these drugs block the absorption of zinc, and it may be possible that these drugs hinder the absorption of other vital nutrients, allowing the body to become depleted. This would make for ideal circumstances for candida to thrive. It could be that the benzodiazepines (in common with the drugs mentioned earlier) raise blood glucose levels, providing more "food" for candida. Many (nondiabetic) users who measured their blood glucose levels found that the blood glucose levels were abnormally high after taking their medication and dropped below normal when the next dose was due. Cimetidine lowers gastric acid secretions and therefore produces an ideal environment for candida growth.

Nondrug Antifungal Substances

Garlic: Nature's Wonder Cure

Garlic is an extremely potent fungicide. It is highly recommended for the treatment of candida and many other health problems. During the 19th century people largely turned away from the use of natural remedies prepared from plants, minerals, and animals, and turned to the use of synthetic drugs. Prior to that people used garlic to cure a wide range of ailments: fevers, chest infections, infected wounds, parasitic infections, and venomous bites. It was also used for kidney problems and stomach ulcers.

The Roman historian Pliny the Elder observed Greek doctors using garlic and recorded:

> *It is good for increasing the flow of urine. The best time to eat*
> *it is when one is about to drink too much, or when one is*

drunk. Garlic boiled or roasted is a diuretic, and relaxes the
stomach. Garlic causes flatulence, because it stops flatulence.

The last statement may be a reference to what we now know as the homeopathic principle of like curing like. Or it may be that eating foods that create gas in the intestines increases the pressure in the bowel. That increased pressure carries away all the pre-existing gas before it, allowing the trapped gas to be expelled.

Modern research has now confirmed that not only did the historical applications of garlic prove correct, but that garlic is a powerful "medicine" for much that ails our technologically advanced, polluted, toxic, drug-orientated, 20th-century world. Garlic has been found to be antibacterial, antifungal, anticarcinogenic, and to be of great benefit to the circulatory system. It also lowers cholesterol levels. Since it is such a powerful cleanser it detoxifies the body, eliminating drug residues and environmental pollutants. Chronic cystitis sufferers have found that regular use of garlic completely clears their symptoms and obviates the need for antibiotics. Some people find garlic also relieves depression and supplies the body with increased energy. In addition to cleansing the body, garlic is a useful source of trace minerals such as copper, iron, selenium, and zinc.

Garlic is effective against a wide range of bacterial, fungal, and parasitic infections. (Even the fumes from freshly pressed garlic can kill fungus grown on a Petri dish in the laboratory.) It kills off the harmful organisms in the gut, protects against the toxins produced, and unlike antibiotics, encourages the growth of helpful organisms. In addition, it aids digestion.

Dr. Susan Minney, in an article titled "Investigation of Anticandidal Activity of Calcium and Magnesium caprylate," writes:

> *If the active antibacterial compounds within the garlic pow-*
> *der were isolated then, weight for weight, their potency*
> *would be very similar to most antibiotics.*
>
> *Garlic has distinct advantages over antibiotics in that its side*
> *effects are very minimal or absent and also that bacteria have*
> *not shown any tendency to become resistant to dried garlic.*

*In summary, the use of dried garlic should be seriously con-
sidered in the treatment, or part treatment, of subacute, non-
life threatening, or chronic bacterial infections, e.g. sore
throats, bronchitis, cystitis, skin infections, boils, gastroenteritis, and diarrhea. It is probable that the use of garlic in life
threatening, acute bacterial diseases will always be secondary
to antibiotics.*

USING FRESH GARLIC

Fresh garlic is an inexpensive and safe way to treat candida overgrowth. Its drawbacks are, of course, the antisocial effects, and, for
some people, the taste. If you (or your family) find these too much to
bear you can use one of the "deodorized" commercial preparations,
but note that the pills must contain the active ingredient *allicin* to be
an effective fungicide. Most garlic pearls have lost allicin during the
manufacturing process. Health food stores stock garlic products but
the quality can be variable. Check with an expert before buying one.

To use fresh garlic, crush one clove (a segment of the bulb) and immediately take it mixed with yogurt, milk, mashed vegetables, or in
olive oil poured on a salad. Wash down the clove with plenty of
water. You may feel a burning sensation or feel slightly sick for a
minute, but this soon passes and is replaced by a feeling of warmth
and, for some, well-being. Do this three times daily, with food or after
eating. Garlic can also be absorbed through the skin. For a fascinating
history of the use of garlic and how to prepare inhalations, and exter-
nal remedies see *Garlic: Nature's Original Remedy*, by Stephen Fulder
and John Blackwood (Inner Traditions) or *Garlic: The Natural Remedy*
by Karen Evennett (Ulysses Press).

JULIA

*Julia was, in her words, "in a state." She had recurrent yeast
infections and cystitis; her face was bloated and covered with
blemishes. Every few weeks she developed a cold, or mouth
ulcers and cold sores on her mouth or inside her nose. She
suffered from weight gain and a persistent rash on her upper
arms and chest. She had a history of taking street drugs and*

abusing alcohol but had been drug-free for two years and only drank on weekends. Her diet was yeast- and sugar-laden and her only exercise was a 15-minute walk to college.

She started on a regimen of garlic therapy. Because she had a plan of action she felt less depressed and after a week on fresh garlic, a clean diet, and exercising more, she could see physical improvements. And her bladder problems disappeared. Three weeks later she was greatly improved; she had lost five pounds, the spots on her face had cleared; the itching and burning in the vulva were gone; and the discharge was much less. She had been using a douche consisting of two crushed garlic cloves to a pint of warm water, straining the garlic water before she used it. She continued taking garlic for six weeks and kept to her new eating plan, with an occasional lapse. The rash on her arms and chest improved over the months, but did not finally clear until she used a prescribed cream. Within three months she felt like "a totally new person."

Julia's story illustrates how discouraging it is to work hard to be drug-free and then to be confronted by a new set of problems. There is very little information available about what can happen in the body after withdrawal from street drugs or when some medications are reduced or withdrawn.

JOHN

John had suffered from a bowel infection while traveling in India a year earlier. He complained of feeling lethargic and bloated and he'd lost his appetite. More recently a rash around his genitals had developed. Hospital tests had been negative. He was in the middle of a three-week colon cleanse that had given him diarrhea, but he knew that was a temporary problem.

John was a vegetarian and did not like sweet foods so his diet needed little adjusting. He took three cloves of raw garlic daily, and, in addition, often cooked with it in his meals. He increased the protein in his diet and took yeast-free nutritional supplements. Within a month he felt stronger. Even though he was still bloated he was not as uncomfortable and his appetite had improved. His energy returned and the fungal rash cleared with sea bathing and sunshine.

John's experience highlights the fact that when you are using garlic, the precise nature of the infection does not really matter because it deals with pathogenic bacteria, fungi, or parasites. Whether it was a candida overgrowth due to a stressed immune system or whether it was a parasite he had picked up on his travels, garlic played an important role in his cure.

GARLIC INTOLERANCE

Many people cannot tolerate garlic. If you know you cannot tolerate any food in the onion family then garlic treatment is probably not for you. However, if it merely gives you gas and you don't have other signs of intolerance such as palpitations, headache, or muscle pains, be patient and your digestive system will get used to it.

Caprylic Acid

This fatty acid is a component of certain food fats that have been included in diets for centuries. It works selectively to inhibit the growth of yeasts, leaving lactobaccillus unharmed. Large quantities are found in breast milk. Commercial preparations are made from coconut oil and are available in most health food stores. Products containing caprylic acid include Caprystatin from Ecological Formulas and and Capralin from Synergy Plus. Caprylic acid is very effective in treating candida and side effects are rare. However, it should not be used by persons with gastritis, gastric ulceration, or intestinal ulceration.

Herbs

One of the latest antifungal, antibacterial, antiparasitic substances that has antiviral activity is made from grapefruit seed extract. Berberine is present in a number of medicinal plants including goldenseal, oregon grape, and barberry. These plants have been used in the treatment of diarrhea in India and in traditional Chinese medicine for over 3000 years.

Note: **These herbs should not be used during pregnancy**. This is the only contraindication, but if you are intolerant to citrus products you might not want to try these herbs.

The Science of Probiotics

Probiotics is the use of live bacterial supplements to kill off harmful bacteria in the gut and restore health. The benefits of lactobacillus acidophilus have been known since the beginning of the century and it is used as a routine part of nutritional and preventative medicine. Nutritionists believe that many degenerative diseases begin with disturbances in intestinal bacteria. After cleansing, the colon needs to be recolonized with helpful bacteria. Health food stores stock bacterial supplements but these cannot always be relied upon to contain live bacteria. If you are lactose intolerant you should look for a nondairy formula. Some available strains include Bio Bifidus from American Biologics or Eugalan Forte from Bio Nutritional or Kyo-Dophilus from Wakunaga.

Live yogurt will provide you with some helpful organisms, but it is unlikely that this will be enough to recolonize the gut if you have a candida problem.

Homeopathy and Candida

HOW DOES HOMEOPATHY WORK?

At the center of homeopathy is the concept of the "Vital Force." Many world philosophies recognize this unseen energy as *prana*, *ch'i*, or *bioenergy*. In homeopathy, when the body manifests symptoms they are seen as the visible expression of a disturbed "Vital Force"; illness is a dynamic disturbance of the "Vital Force," which must be restored to a full functional harmony. In a healthy individual the "Vital Force" keeps the "clocks wound"; in an unhealthy individual sickness causes the clocks to "wind down" because the immunity is weakened, causing symptoms to develop.

Orthodox medicine, on the other hand, sees symptoms as evidence of a morbid process that must be eradicated or suppressed; it puts great store in the study of pathological change, chemical disturbances, bacteria, and viruses, leading to treatment directed against the symptoms. Conventional medicine treats only the symptoms presented while the homeopath treats the *whole* person.

Take, for instance, five patients with acne. The conventional practitioner will treat all of them similarly; the homeopath, however, may end up prescribing different remedies for each of them because she is treating the *person* as opposed to the *symptoms*. Although they all have acne, the disease has been manifested through different medical backgrounds with varying underlying causes.

The homeopath takes a detailed history, looking at the uniqueness of the individual. The purpose of this close scrutiny is to elicit enough information to paint a picture of the person's lifestyle and being, to enable the homeopath to make a remedy selection appropriate to the *totality* of the person's symptoms. The potency of the remedy that ideally matches the dynamic plane of the disease at that time is then selected. When the remedy and potency have been chosen, this is called the *similimum*; when the patient picture matches the remedy picture progress is almost guaranteed.

THE PRINCIPLES OF HOMEOPATHY

The foundation of homeopathy is *similia similimum curantur*: "Like shall be cured by like," or "That which makes sick shall heal." Samuel Hahnemann, the founder of homeopathy, stated that the matching remedy for a disease is a substance that in a healthy person produces the same symptoms as displayed in the sick person.

- *The single remedy.* All the symptoms are arranged in order of importance and the remedy is given. The principle of the single remedy treating the whole person is in sharp contrast to the allopathic system (traditional western medicine), where often multiple drugs are prescribed at one time.

- *The minimum dose.* Very minute doses of the selected remedy are administered. Hahnemann discovered that by reducing dosages, unwanted aggravations (or side effects) were cut down, and the remedies were still effective. He went on to develop a system of diluting remedies to a point where not a single molecule of the original substance is present, only its energy pattern. He called this process of repeated dilution, along with succussion (shaking), *potentization*. Apparently it is in the succussion that curative properties are released; the higher the potency the smaller the amount of the medicinal substance is present in the solution.

- *Provings.* Substances used for homeopathic remedies come from animal, vegetable, and mineral sources. Their potentially healing properties are tested on healthy persons where there is no risk of the results being tainted by a disease picture.

HOW DOES HOMEOPATHY WORK WITH CANDIDIASIS?

In my experience, candidiasis is best tackled using a dietary approach in conjunction with suitable homeopathic remedy supplements. It is important to stress that although the candidiasis can be fairly easily treated, underlying causes need to be addressed. For example, candidiasis might result from the use of repeated antibiotics for recurring sore throats.

JANE

Jane, a 32-year-old female, had been on the contraceptive pill for nine years. She complained of

- halitosis
- bloating and belching after meals
- proneness to sore throats
- craving sweets and chocolates
- allergies to lanolin and topical alcohol
- migraine headaches induced by strong light
- no energy or stamina
- poor memory
- muscle weakness
- poor, unrefreshing sleep

Progress: Jane showed marked improvement after one month and required further treatment for three months. Homeopathic remedies effectively strengthened her immune system. I felt prolonged exposure to the pill and frequent courses of antibiotics were the culprits.

JOAN

Joan, a 23-year-old female, complained of severe depression for two years. She had been prescribed antidepressants by a psychiatrist. Joan had bouts of recurrent tonsillitis that were treated with antibiotics. She always felt low after treatment. She had a profound lack of energy and wondered if she had ME or severe premenstrual syndrome. Other complaints included

- feeling alone, forsaken, suicidal, weepy—symptoms were worse in morning
- feeling like things were out of focus
- feeling as if she was out of touch with reality
- having no middle moods
- fearing as if something was about to happen
- being easily stressed
- having poor sleep

Progress: Antidepressant drugs were slowly reduced under supervision. After one month she showed a dramatic improvement mentally. It took nine months for her to be symptom free, and now this patient is in control of her life.

According to Elizabeth Edmundson, a homeopathic practitioner who has had an interest in candida problems for many years, homeopathy is a powerful facet of candida treatment because it treats the root cause of the disease; it deals with why the patient initially becomes susceptible to the fungus in the first place, rather than solely treating the candida.

Essential Oils

Before discussing the use of essential oils as a treatment for candida, it must be said that while many of the oils can safely be included in self-help care, they are powerful substances; some are toxic. It is important to follow the instructions of a qualified aromatherapist or only use the oils recommended in aromatherapy books. There are some excellent books on the market that give clear instructions on choosing and mixing oils for everyday problems such as tension, headaches, indigestion, lethargy, anxiety, depression, and so on. *Note: Beauty therapists are only trained to use the oils to promote relaxation and for skin care; they are not trained to use them for specific medicinal effects (aromatherapy).*

The medicinal value of distilled oil from plants, fruit, wood, and resins has been known for thousands of years. During the past 30 years there has been a resurgence of interest in their use and medical research has confirmed that they have great value in alleviating or curing a wide range of physical and emotional conditions. Essential oils can be administered through the skin, through inhalation, or orally.

When mixed with a base or carrier oil they are absorbed through the fatty tissue of the body during massage. A 20-minute soak in the bath in warm water with a few drops of oil allows the same penetration. The vapors enter a primitive part of the brain called the limbic system when they are inhaled from a tissue, in hot water, or from an oil burner. (Tranquilizers also work on this part of the brain.) Except in the case where a book clearly states that the oils can be taken orally— for example, one drop of peppermint oil in a tumbler of warm water for the relief of gas—they should not be taken internally unless prescribed by a qualified aromatherapist.

Many of the oils have bactericidal and fungicidal properties, but the most important essential oil prescribed for the relief of candida is tea tree.

Tea Tree Oil for Candida

For thousands of years the Australian Bundjalung Aborigines have valued the healing properties of the tree *Melaleuca alternifolia*. Research shows that pure tea tree oil is an extremely complex substance containing at least 48 organic compounds that work together in synergy to produce maximum healing benefits.

The first European to collect samples of the leaves was Joseph Banks in 1770. At about the same time Captain Cook's sailors made a "spicy and refreshing tea" from the leaves of the *Melaleuca alternifolia* tree to replace the tea they had brought from England. Hence the name, "Tea Tree."

In 1922, an Australian chemist conducted experiments using the leaves of the *Melaleuca alternifolia* tree and announced his results to the Royal Society of New South Wales. He discovered the very high antiseptic power of the oil: 13 times stronger than the carbolic acid that was used as an antiseptic at the time. His findings prompted additional research and in 1930, under the heading of "A New Australian Germicide," the editor of the *Medical Journal of Australia* reported on the use of the oil in general practice.

The results, obtained under a variety of conditions, were most encouraging. One striking feature was that the oil dissolved pus and left the surfaces of infected wounds clean so that its germicidal action became more effective without any apparent damage to the tissue. In 1930, the *British Medical Journal* stated: "The oil is a powerful disinfectant, but it is non-poisonous and non-irritant, and has been used successfully in a very wide range of septic conditions."

Although it was found to be effective in many conditions, including fungal skin problems, demand outstripped production and synthetic germicides were developed. With the advent of miracle drugs, starting with synthetic penicillin, the value of tea tree was overlooked.

In the 1970s, there was renewed interest in the oil and it is now available in a wide range of products world-wide. Tea tree oil can effectively treat a great number of ailments due to its healing and infection-fighting properties. These include athlete's foot, toenail infection, acne and dermatitis, mouth ulcers and cold sores, and a number of other complaints associated with candida and fungal infections. Its value in treating yeast infection and cystitis is described on page 12. You will find tea tree oil in stores that stock essential oils.

CHAPTER SEVEN

Diet

It is impossible to create a candida diet that would suit everyone. There are so many approaches to diets for the control of candidiasis that if you have read a few books on the subject you are probably totally confused. Some practitioners insist on very strict regimes. Others say keep to a diet and if you have an odd lapse take an extra dose of your antifungal substance. Others say don't worry too much if you are on anti-candida medication, eat what you like. (The latter, in my opinion, is going too far because a cure would take forever.) Before you get discouraged by the idea of a restricted diet remember that there are other ways (see page 26 on desensitization) to deal with candida, although you are unlikely to recover from any condition if you abuse your body with junk food and excessive alcohol.

The Right Diet for You

Your personal choice will be determined by your likes and dislikes, the severity of your symptoms, how desperate you are for them to disappear, food intolerance, and how much stress is involved in your sticking to a rigid diet. This chapter offers two plans: a fairly strict anti-candida diet and a more relaxed eating plan. In Part II of the book a stricter diet plan is offered.

Diet as a Medicine, Not a Punishment

You might choose to follow the stricter diet for the first three weeks and then go on the more relaxed diet. (However, I believe that staying on very restricted diets for long periods should be avoided not only because of the danger of your intake being nutritionally narrow, but because eating should be a pleasure and not a continual worry. Practitioners helping people with candida and allergy problems have become increasingly aware of what I call "Candida/Allergy Diet Neurosis." Some people are so obsessed by what they can't eat that their diet becomes too narrow and they become malnourished; this affects their immune and nervous systems. Relax, be balanced, have the odd treat, rotate your foods, watch your weight and above all understand that dietary adjustments are a temporary medicine to clean the digestive tract and help your immune system.

Approach the candida diet not as a life sentence to a strange diet, but as a temporary change to improve your health. After the first month you can have the odd lapse and then as your symptoms disappear, you can look forward to a normal healthy way of eating. Diets laden with refined sugars and fats are dangerous, even for those without candida, so hopefully you will never go back to eating in that fashion. In fact, it is unlikely that you will want to after you have experienced the difference in your well-being while you have been eating healthily. Be kind to yourself, particularly if you have been eating carbohydrates or drinking excessively for comfort. You also might feel anxiety or grief at having to give up your "security blankets." So often the cry is "but I cannot live without bread!" But you *can* give up the food that is making you ill, and you *will* if it is necessary for you to get better.

The following are guidelines to starve the candida:

- Buy absolutely fresh foods
- Do not eat refined carbohydrates
- Restrict unrefined carbohydrates

- Aim for a diet as low as possible in yeast

- Avoid or cut down on foods that contain antibiotics or steroids

Overripe fruit, limp vegetables, and bread that has been around for a few days all harbor mold spores. If possible, shop for smaller quantities from stores that have a rapid turnover of produce. Take extra care in storing food; wash out the bread bin regularly or store bread in refrigerator. If you are using only small quantities, slice a loaf as soon as you buy it and freeze it. You can take your portion out daily: it defrosts quickly or can be toasted.

Diet One: A Moderate Approach

AVOID OR CUT DOWN ON

- sugar, white or brown

- molasses, sucrose, glucose, dextrose, jam

- white flour and all products made from white flour: cakes, cookies, etc.

- all processed grains, including some prepared breakfast cereals

- yeasty foods: hard cheese, blue cheese, brewer's yeast, or any supplements containing yeast

- vinegar, carbonated drinks, and all fermented products such as alcohol

- dried fruit

- canned fruit in syrup

YOU CAN EAT

- whole grains: whole-grain bread, pasta, brown rice, any other unrefined grains

- puffed wheat, puffed rice, shredded wheat, muesli or homemade muesli—all sugar-free

- meat, poultry, eggs

- dairy products: milk, cream, butter, cottage cheese, soft cheeses, yogurt (preferably plain or nonfat)
- fish—fresh or canned
- legumes: lentils, peas, beans, chickpeas
- nuts and seeds
- spices
- fresh or dried herbs
- large quantities of raw or steamed vegetables
- useful thickeners for soups and stews: arrowroot; grated potatoes; additive-free vegetable stock; marigold, available from health-food stores
- fresh fruit
- olive oil, any other vegetable oil, margarine
- all-fruit jam
- diet drinks (in moderation)
- fructose (fruit sugar), honey (in moderation)
- dry white wine

Diet Two: A Stricter Approach

You could begin with the following diet for three weeks to get a good start on starving the candida, or before starting antifungal drugs/substances. This would minimize the die off symptoms.

BANNED FOODS

- sugar (white or brown), molasses, sucrose, glucose, dextrose, or any product containing sugar
- white flour and all products made from white flour: cakes, bread, cookies, etc.
- pasta, white rice
- all prepared breakfast cereals

- cured products: bacon, smoked salmon, other smoked fish
- all fermented products, vinegar, pickles, chutney, sauerkraut, tofu, soy sauce
- alcohol
- tea, coffee, cocoa, Ovaltine
- any malted product
- all dairy products: milk, cheese, cottage cheese (with the possible exception of live plain yogurt)
- mushrooms, truffles
- dried fruit
- fresh fruit for the first three weeks
- spices, dried herbs
- canned foods
- artificial sweeteners, diet drinks
- nuts
- citric acid
- cream of tartar

You Can Eat

- restricted whole grains: up to 80 grams per day (one small slice of whole-grain bread = 30 grams)
- brown rice, Ryvita, rye bread, rice cakes, oat cakes, whole oats, millet, buckwheat, barley
- whole-wheat pasta, whole-wheat noodles, buckwheat pasta
- eggs, free-range chicken, turkey, duck, rabbit, lamb, venison, fresh fish, shellfish
- legumes: peas, beans, lentils, chickpeas, etc.
- seeds: sunflower, sesame, linseed, pumpkin
- all raw or cooked vegetables (eat mountains of them)
- sea vegetables

Why Some Foods Are Banned

All the foods on the formidable "banned" list either feed candida or contain additives that chronic sufferers react to. The powdery bloom on some fruits is mold, and nuts and spices often harbor mold. Some nutritionists ban artificial sweeteners because some of them are made from sugar (NutraSweet and saccharin are not) and they believe that their inclusion in the diet perpetuates a craving for sugar.

Note: Some lifelong tea and coffee drinkers have no trouble abstaining; others have what is known as the "Caffeine Storm." This happens when all the caffeine in the body is mobilized and before it is eliminated, causing severe headaches, nausea, and aches and pains. A cup of tea or coffee usually eases the symptoms within half an hour. If this happens to you, phase tea and coffee out gradually.

Sugar

You do not need sugar for energy. On the contrary, it can drain your energy. Sugar offers not only empty calories, it is the food of choice for candida, and it prevents the absorption of essential minerals and vitamins as well. It also plays havoc with your blood-sugar levels and disrupts the function of your pancreas, causing a multitude of unpleasant symptoms including panic attacks.

Sugar in tea or coffee should be stopped immediately. You will get used to it eventually and if it makes you cut down on tea and coffee, so much the better. Try not to turn to regular use of artificial sweeteners; this just prolongs the desire for sweet drinks. Occasional use of sweeteners or a diet soft drink can be regarded as a treat. Withdrawal or sugar craving cause some people to abandon the candida diet. If you think you are in danger of doing this use very small amounts of fructose (fruit sugar, available from pharmacies and health food stores) or honey. These do not disturb the pancreas and are less likely to trigger yeast growth. Look for honey from bees that have not been fed sugar. Organic honey is best but there may be brands that are less expensive.

There are some useful yeast- /sugar-free cookbooks on the market.

Refined Carbohydrates (Sugar and Starches)

All refined grains and products made from refined grains encourage yeast growth. They have also lost many essential nutrients during processing. Diets high in refined starches are the main cause of the Toxic Colon Syndrome. The starch combines with mucus in the gut and forms a gluey layer that collects on the bowel wall. The effects of this have been described earlier. There is little argument about the inclusion of refined carbohydrates in the diet: most practitioners recommend their avoidance, except perhaps when someone with a wheat intolerance finds white bread, particularly toasted, less of a problem.

Diet Drinks

Some people imagine because diet drinks are sugar-free (check labels because some sweeteners are sugar-based) that it is okay to drink a large bottle daily. However, because you are trying to clean chemicals and additives from your system this does not seem like a good idea. In addition, all soft drinks contain citric acid, which encourages yeast growth and can also make cystitis sufferers very uncomfortable. You could make your own soft drinks from freshly squeezed fruit juice and carbonated mineral water.

Dairy Products

There is a division of opinion on dairy products. Some practitioners recommend them, particularly for underweight people, and believe lactic acid is helpful in dealing with candida problems; others discourage their use. Dairy products are mucus-forming and it would be well to avoid them if you have chest or coughing problems, if you are intolerant to them, or if you are on a colon-cleansing program. Otherwise, go by how you feel in deciding whether to include them.

Eggs

It is a pity that eggs have had such bad press lately. Egg yolks are rich in essential nutrients and also help to keep the bowel flora healthy. If you are not in a high-risk heart disease group, and if you use eggs as part of a healthy diet, their cholesterol content is not a problem. A well-cooked egg is a useful addition to the anti-candida diet. Try to use free-range eggs, which do not contain antibiotics.

Complex or Unrefined Carbohydrates

Whole grains retain all their nutrients, and because their fiber content has not been discarded, they give the stool bulk and stimulate peristalsis (the contractions and movements in the bowel), thereby keeping the bowel clean. Complex carbohydrates are broken down slowly in the body and release a steady flow of glucose into the blood that prevents the "kangarooing" of blood glucose levels, with its resultant drop in energy and craving for sugary foods. There is a division of opinion on whether to restrict complex carbohydrates. Some practitioners say eat as much as you wish of any whole grain you can tolerate. Others restrict them, saying that they still encourage fungal growth even if they are unrefined.

Will Changing My Diet Affect Me?

It could, particularly if you have been accustomed to a highly refined carbohydrate menu. You might experience withdrawal symptoms, including sugar cravings. Change of diet and/or the addition of supplements can also produce lethargy and aches and pains in the first few weeks. Be prepared for this and welcome it: it can be the candida dying off or the effect of other toxins being released from the body.

Nutritional Supplements

Many people have commented that they are bewildered by rows of supplements in health food stores. The following information is a guide to help you choose ones that help to build the immune system. If the choice and dosage differs from those suggested by your doctor or nutritionist be guided by them because they will have more knowledge about your individual needs. If you find you cannot take supplements at the suggested dosages build up to the full dosage slowly or take them two or three times a week if that is all you can manage. Remember that supplements should be regarded as a medicine to correct deficiencies and as such should be taken as a course, not indefinitely, unless this has been advised by your doctor or nutritionist. Follow the instructions on the bottle carefully and keep them out of the reach of children. Be sure to get good quality supplements.

Penny Davenport, a nutritional therapist, recommends the following:

VITAMINS

- Vitamin A (as beta carotene)
- B complex (single B vitamins should always be taken with the complex to ensure balance)
- Biotin (prevents the yeast from becoming invasive, often comes with folic acid)
- Vitamin C (as a sustained release formula or in small divided doses; antiviral and immune boosting)

MINERALS, ENZYMES, AND OTHERS

- Zinc (elemental form)
- Selenium (inhibits free radical damage; boosts the immune system; and is strongly antifungal)
- Kelp (all essential trace minerals; excellent for balancing the thyroid gland, which often contributes to a low immune system)
- Magnesium (taken in the morning, helps muscle ache and fatigue)
- Probiotics (as well as Bifido bacteria and acidophilus, Lactobacillus Salivarius is also available; it digests protein molecules that have not been completely digested, a common cause of autotoxicity.)
- Digestive enzymes (incompletely digested food causes many problems; there are now a variety of vegetarian formulas available in vegetable gelatin)
- Anti-parasite formula (grapefruit seed concentrated extract; many candida sufferers are found to have parasites)

HERBS

- Garlic (highly antifungal and promotes the growth of probiotic organisms)
- Echinacea (stimulates production of white blood cells)
- Artemesia, Barberry, Pulsatilla, and Zingiber combined with grapefruit extract are antibiotic, antifungal, and antiparasitic
- Chinese herbs shizandra, acanthopanax, and astragalus (boost immunity)
- Pau d'Arco tea (boosts the immune system, and strongly antifungal)

ESSENTIAL FATTY ACIDS

- Gamma Linoleic Acid and Evening Primrose Oil (essential to produce balanced hormones, prostaglandins; one function is to keep yeast cells at bay, and to stimulate the immunity gland, the thymus, to produce T-cells)

Because supplements are expensive, it is important to know which ones to choose and to find ways of being economical. For instance, vitamin C is essential and the powder is the cheapest form to buy it in. If you buy it buffered with minerals it costs a little extra. Herbs are always economical and making a tisane (an herbal infusion or tea) is simple. Because they boost the immune system and are antifungal (and in some cases antiparasitic), the combinations can be useful. With probiotics, try the cheaper ones first to see if they work for you. Sometimes it makes more sense to take less of a quality concentrated form.

A good all-round concentrate that gives a wide range of essential nutrients is freshwater algae such as Spirulina. If you cannot find one or your health food store does not stock the items you want, there are excellent mail order companies who also specialize in giving advice.

If you are on a limited income, you must stick to the diet before investing in supplements. It is not expensive. Think what you would save on your normal shopping bill: no bread, cookies, cakes, tea, coffee, soft drinks, dairy products, not to mention candy and chocolate. All this leaves plenty of money for a variety of vegetables. Never go hungry, eat small meals regularly. And remember to drink lots of water.

CHAPTER EIGHT

Looking After Yourself

Taking care of your general health is a vital part of the anti-candida program. Stimulating the circulatory and lymphatic systems by exercising and getting plenty of fresh air and sunlight are valuable components in conquering *candida albicans*. Getting a good night sleep is also essential.

The Lymphatic System

This system is part of the body's defense against disease. A clear, watery fluid that contains white blood cells called lymph, which relies on muscle contraction for its circulation, is carried through a complex network of small vessels and carries cellular refuse (bacteria and certain proteins) on the way. The waste is then passed into the bloodstream where it is processed.

The lymphatic system does not have a pump (unlike the blood circulation that has the heart) so when you don't move the lymph slows down. The result can be fluid retention, causing the cells that rely on lymph for their nourishment to become malnourished. This is why exercise is critical to your well-being. Even if you have to stay in bed for some reason you can help circulate the lymphatic system by gently squeezing each group of muscles in your body in turn, and by rotating your ankles and wrists. Massage can also be very helpful.

Exercise

It is often hard to convince people that exercise is an important part of recovery from most conditions. There is a general misconception that because you feel ill you should be as inactive as possible. If you do not have a fever, inflamed muscles, or any condition likely to be adversely affected by exercise, then move. You will delay your recovery if you don't. Build up the amount of exercise you do slowly; it is unwise to start vigorous activities if you have been sedentary for months. You will see below why exercise is so important. (Check with your physician before you start on an exercise program or if you are unsure whether your condition warrants bed rest.)

Inactivity affects your circulation and as a consequence, your organic functions. For example, inactivity causes your digestive system to become sluggish; this results in constipation. Muscles are also affected, not only because they are improperly nourished, but by a build-up of crystals formed from the waste products of digestion. This build-up can cause generalized aches and pains as well as local tender spots. If you don't move your body, the crystals cannot be dispersed. Tension also locks these crystals into the muscles. A vicious circle begins: a build-up in the shoulder area can be very painful, which in turn causes you to move less.

In addition, if you do not move the muscles in your neck and shoulders you restrict the blood supply to your head, creating endless problems. Ask yourself how much you are holding yourself back by sitting long hours in a car, at a desk, or even watching television without moving. Your brain can become sluggish, too. When full circulation is restored symptoms of anxiety and depression can be dramatically relieved. Building simple stretching exercises into your daily life, or a brisk walk in your lunchtime break, take little time and help. But to feel the real benefits of exercise you have to incorporate more vigorous movement into your daily life.

Aerobic Exercise

Aerobic exercise is a form of physical conditioning that enhances circulatory or respiratory performance and consists of sustained, vigorous exercise. It utilizes the long, smooth muscles of the upper legs and arms, which pump blood (and lymphatic fluid) to the heart and liver, and to the lungs for cleansing and oxygenating. This boosts the immune system by encouraging regeneration and white blood cell replacement. Aerobic exercise also stimulates the production of serotonin (a sleep precursor) and endorphins (which are pleasure giving and pain relieving). And of great importance, aerobic exercise strengthens the muscles of the heart and increases the capacity of the lungs.

For aerobic exercise to be effective it needs to be done for 20 minutes, 3 times a week, at a pace that makes you breathe deeply and hard, but not causing you to be out of breath. It should be an effort, but not exhausting. (You should be able to talk as you exercise.) A target heart-rate range must be sustained for 20 minutes. Good examples of aerobic exercise include swimming, walking, gentle jogging, running, cycling, and step and aerobic classes.

Water Therapies

Caution: Consult your doctor before using water treatments if you have heart trouble, raised blood pressure, diabetes, epilepsy or have any condition that might be aggravated by temperature extremes. If you are on medication, particularly tranquilizers, it is also advisable to check with your doctor.

Hydrotherapy

Hydrotherapy has been used in spas for thousands of years. One treatment, the *sitzbath*, immerses parts of the body in different temperatures. You sit in hot water with your feet in cold water for three minutes, then reverse for one minute. The result is quite dramatic: a glowing sensation that you feel down the entire length of the spine. Sitzbaths also boost the immune system and circulation in the abdominal organs, a good treatment for candida.

It is not easy to have a proper sitzbath without special plumbing, but you can improvise with a bathtub, two buckets, and a baby bath. It can also be done with two baby baths.

1. Sit in a bathtub of hot water with your feet in a bucket of cold water. The hot water around the bucket will raise the temperature of the cold water, so keep the water cold with an ice pack or a plastic bottle two-thirds full of water that has been frozen. After three minutes get out. Lift out the cold bucket and change.

2. Next, sit in a baby bath of cold water and put your feet in a bucket of hot water. After one minute change again.

3. Sit in the hot water for another three minutes. Make sure the water in the bathtub is still hot. You will not get the same effect with tepid water.

4. Change from sitting in the hot water to cold water at least three times. This might seem like a lot of effort but the effect is worth it. Alternating hot and cold showers are also invigorating, but do not have the same dramatic lift.

Sea Bathing and Walking in the Sand

The tonic effect of sea bathing is well known, and being at the sea-shore has an added benefit. Walking ankle deep in the sea boosts your circulation and can be very soothing for your nervous system. Tension can be discharged through the soles of the feet because they are massaged by the sand. It is similar to the effect reflexology has on the body.

Mineral Baths

Seaweed, mud, herb, and essential oil baths all have detoxifying and healing properties and can promote relaxation.

The skin is the largest organ in the body. While the digestive tract and the kidneys are the main organs of excretion, the skin also plays a very important role in cleansing the body. If it is kept healthy it can be a wonderful waste-disposal system. During the past one hundred years the popularity of *hydrotherapy* has waned; people turned away from such natural healing methods and moved toward drug treatments, sometimes with disastrous results.

A fever is nature's way of helping us to lose toxins through the skin. Some water therapies simulate a fever by inducing sweating. Steam baths, saunas, and jacuzzis encourage detoxification of the body through the skin.

Salt baths encourage detoxification and greatly help muscle and joint pains. Add 2 pounds of salt or three cups full of Epsom salts to a comfortably hot bath and lie in it for 20 minutes; add hot water as it cools. If you drink a cup of peppermint tea or a pint of hot water with juice from half a lemon and a teaspoonful of honey while you soak it will further encourage sweating. An ice pack or cold wash cloth on your forehead will make you feel more comfortable.

If you wrap up in warm towels or a cotton sheet and get into a warm bed you should perspire freely and sleep well. If you have to bathe during the day, finish with a cold shower and rest for half an hour. You could do this three times a week.

You could have a foot bath while reading or watching television. It helps stimulate your circulation and eases aching feet. Alternate tubs of hot and cold water, keeping your feet in the tub for two minutes each for a period of about 20 minutes. If you wish, add one cup of salt or half a cup of Epsom salts to the hot water and an ice pack to the cold tub. When you have finished, wrap your feet in a towel and rest.

Exercises in the water or swimming also stimulate the lymphatic system and rids the body of toxins.

Swimming

Swimming stimulates the immune system and has been shown to elevate mood levels. Allergy sufferers may not want to swim in chlorinated pools.

Skin Brushing

Not exactly water therapy, but related, skin brushing is a good way to stimulate your lymphatic system. It involves brushing all over with a natural bristle brush for about ten minutes before your shower or bath. You can also use a loofa in the bath or shower. Start with the soles of your feet and brush all areas of the body except broken skin, the face, neck, and breasts. It can be boring but the results are worth it. In addition to eliminating toxins by increasing circulation, it will also improve the texture of your skin. The Body Shop and many health food stores and pharmacies have skin brushes and loofas. You might have an old hairbrush that would do the job, but be sure to wash it carefully.

Sunlight, Air, and Daylight

The exposure to sunlight, fresh air, and daylight are fundamental considerations when striving for better health, and the avoidance of *candida albicans*. Sunlight has numerous positive effects on your health. It has been shown that it kills bacteria and fungus on the skin; short exposure to ultraviolet light, either directly from the sun or from a sun bed, can help to eradicate fungal skin infections. Another benefit of sunlight is the production of vitamin D. However, baking in the sun or overdoing tanning treatments ages the skin and can lead to skin cancer, so moderate the use of sunbathing as a treatment.

Fresh air and proper breathing are also basic ingredients to creating an environment that nourishes overall good health. Unless people actually have chest problems, it is often difficult to convince them of the benefits of good breathing habits. It is even harder to impress upon them the dangers of continually filling their lungs with stale air. However, it has been shown that exposure to fresh air kills fungus. Candida sufferers should avoid being in dank, moldy places such as cellars and damp rooms because fungus needs damp, moist areas to survive and propagate. In the same vein, those with chemical intolerance should avoid paint fumes, being near photocopiers, and being exposed to the myriad other chemical pollutants.

And finally, in order to maintain good health and normal brain functioning, it is essential that you are exposed to a certain amount of daylight. You should expose yourself to daylight for a minimum of 20 minutes, preferably in the brightest part of the day. Staying indoors when you are depressed or ill only compounds your problems. Even if you are severely agoraphobic you could sit at an open window without your glasses.

For further reading on these subjects read *Anxiety & Depression: A Natural Approach* (Ulysses Press).

Electrical Pollution

The immune system can also be affected by environments contaminated by low-level radiation from electrical equipment and from an overload of positive ions in the atmosphere. If ventilation is poor and you walk on synthetic carpets, wear synthetic clothes, and are surrounded by plastic furniture you are unlikely to feel good at the end of the day. Electrically polluted air can be the cause not only of respiratory problems but of headaches, irritability, digestive problems, and depression.

Ions are the electrically charged particles in the air around us that we breathe in and absorb through the skin. Ideally, there should be a balance between the positive and negative particles. If the air is overloaded with positively charged particles it can have a powerful effect on the nervous system. If this happens the brain overproduces the chemical serotonin, which can lead to nasal congestion, lethargy, feeling sticky (not the same feeling as being too hot), and swollen. Before a storm there is an excess of positive ions; for many this creates an oppressive, restless feeling—like being "under the weather." After a thunderstorm the air is negatively charged. It is then that everything smells fresh and we experience "the calm after the storm"; our energy returns and our mood improves. Some people are more affected by ions than others, in the same way that some people are more irritable and restless when the moon is full, and others are not.

Negative ions have a tonic effect on the nervous system and reduce histamine levels in the blood. Not only does negative ionization clean the air and kill bacteria and viruses, it can be used in the treatment of other medical conditions such as asthma, bronchitis, and migraine headaches. Candida sufferers, particularly if they have allergies, would do well to use an ionizer in their bedrooms; some people have ionizers in every room. (They are also available for use in a car.) A feeling of well-being can also be attained by breathing the air by the sea, waterfalls, flowing water, even the air in the shower, because it is negatively charged. You cannot overdose on negative ions; you can breathe in as many as you like.

The State of the Electromagnetic Field

We are electrical beings: our hearts, brains, muscles, and nerves produce a subtle form of electricity. This electricity discharges around our bodies and forms an electromagnetic field, our aura. In the 1930s, a pair of Russian electricians, V.K. and S.D. Kirlian, developed a form of photography that was able to display this field. It was then determined that all living things are surrounded by these fields.

A leading modern researcher on electromagnetic pollution, Dr. Robert O. Becker, author of *The Body Electric*, believes that human-made electromagnetic fields from power lines and electrical appliances can cause depression, a depressed immune system, and other health problems. The influence on one's whole being—body, mind, and soul—of the electromagnetic field is dismissed by many scientists and considered to be mystical nonsense. This is unfortunate because some scientists relying on Kirlian photography, believe that disease is manifested in the electromagnetic field before physical symptoms appear.

Some believe that balancing areas of low energy by working on the electromagnetic field could be the medicine of the future. This is not new; similarities can be found in ancient forms of Chinese healing.

A modern pioneer in this field is Dolores Kreiger, a nurse who developed the technique therapeutic touch, which clears and energizes the electromagnetic field. It is taught in some nursing schools and is explained in her book *Therapeutic Touch: How To Use Your Hands to*

Help or Heal (Simon & Schuster). Janet Macrae, one of Dolores Krei-ger's students, has written a book, *Therapeutic Touch: A Practical Guide* (Knopf), that anyone can use. (Do not worry if you do not feel the various qualities of the energies she describes when you are treating either yourself or other people. Don't try to fit someone else's experi-ence into your own; your hands are unique.)

CAN I FEEL MY OWN ELECTRICAL FIELD?

Only 1 percent of people of the people who have tried to feel their own electrical field can't. Go ahead, try it. You might have to try a few times before you can be sure, but the more you practice the more sensitive your hands will become. There are several ways to build up the energy in your hands before you use them. Here is a simple method I saw given at a workshop by Julie Soskin, a specialist in the field of personal and spiritual growth:

Breathe in slowly and visualize yourself being filled with Universal Energy, *prana, ch'i,* or whatever you wish to call it.

Increasing the energy between your hands:

1. Hold your arms out in front of you, raising one about a foot above the other.

2. Clench and release your fists rapidly for about 15 sec-onds.

3. Lower the raised hand and raise the other; repeat the fist clenching and releasing.

4. Keeping your arms out in front: repeat steps 2 and 3.

5. Relax your shoulders: point your fingers upward as if you were going to clap. Make an accordion movement with your hands, in and out, just a few inches, but do not bring your palms into contact.

You will feel a resistance or a feeling of pressure, heat, or tingling between your hands. Some people say they feel as if there is foam rubber between their palms, others describe feelings of tingling, throbbing, or pulling.

USING YOUR HANDS TO CLEAR THE ELECTROMAGNETIC FIELD

Now that your hands are energized you can use them to clear positive ions from your immediate environment, relieve headaches and nasal congestion, increase relaxation, and ease discomfort in muscles and joints.

To do this:

1. Rub your feet and massage under the arch for about one minute. If your feet are very tense take a little longer over them, then place them flat on the floor if you are sitting.

2. Sit relaxed or lie on the floor or bed; slow down your breathing.

3. Close your eyes and imagine yourself totally well and peaceful. If you cannot attain this image, give yourself the command, "I am totally well and peaceful," and imagine that a pure white light is entering your head, filling your body, and then exiting from your fingers and palms. Reach up beyond your head and stroke about three to four inches above your body just as though you were touching it; then down over your face, neck, chest, and abdomen. Next sweep your hands to either side of the body. This is important because you need to take the congestion away from your body. You will feel prickling or heat in your hands as you pick up congestion. You can just flick this off as though you are shaking water from your hands.

4. Continue stroking for about ten minutes or until your arms feel tired.

5. Now, as you continue to imagine that you are filled with white light, that you see it coming from your hands, hold your hands over your abdomen and imagine your digestive tract and all your internal organs becoming healthy and vitalized.

INCREASING ENERGY IN SELECTED AREAS

In this part of the exercise you are sending energy to an area of discomfort, perhaps an infected vagina or bloated abdomen. You may feel heat or cold and possibly rumblings in your gut. Don't be surprised if it makes loud noises. This is just a sign that you are relaxing. As you practice this you will get a feeling of being finished. That is the only way to describe the sensation of an area having taken enough energy. You might also have noticed your nose feeling less congested or your sinuses making popping noises when you were working around your head. You can transfer energy in the same way to any aching muscles or joints that you can reach. Clearing congestion from the field also helps to cool a fever, ease itching, and reduce swelling.

Many people are very enthusiastic about therapeutic touch and are eager to use it to help others. This is certainly to be encouraged, but it should not be attempted before you are well and have learned more about it. There are people who teach this technique, which is sometimes called "auric massage."

The Inner Child, the Spirit

This might appear to be a strange conclusion to a section of a book about parasitic yeast, but since I believe that total health is dependent on the harmony of body, mind, and spirit, I feel the need to include, with humility, the little I have learned in my own emotional and spiritual struggle.

Parasitic Emotions

Negative feelings about ourselves—anger, a lack of self-worth, a lack of self-love, a failure to see our place in the world—and fears, particularly the fear of death, can continually eat away at our "life force," preventing us from living in the here and now. These feelings and fears can disrupt our lives as much as yeast overgrowths in our gut, or any other physical problem.

How Can I Love Myself?

Ask yourself:

- Am I crying inside?
- Am I lonely, even in midst of company?

- Am I hyperventilating?

- Am I addicted to something, such as gambling or alcohol?

- Am I judgmental?

- Do I continually criticize the behavior of others?

- Do I blame others, my life circumstances, the world, for my feelings?

- Am I always looking for a tomorrow that never comes?

- Do I continually look to others for approval?

- Have I incorporated the negative feelings people have or have had about me? My mother/father/siblings/teachers/employers/partners?

- Am I afraid?

- Am I so afraid of fear itself that I can't face why I am afraid?

- Am I afraid to express anger?

- Does my anger come out in inappropriate places? Do I take my anger out on the people I know will take my anger and still love me? Do I take my anger out on strangers for whom I do not risk losing love?

- Am I afraid to love—even myself?

Self-love, which is very different from narcissism and selfishness, takes a lot of practice and awareness. M. Scott Peck in his book *The Road Less Traveled* covers this subject in depth with wisdom and love. It is important to be open to the possibility that you are not meeting your own needs and need to find a counselor, psychotherapist, or even a friend to support you while you explore this area.

Where do these feelings come from and why do we hang on to them? They come from our life experience (beginning prenatally). And we are often reluctant to give them up because we will have to confront them head on. Most of us shy away from this confrontation out of fear, or perhaps because we lack the insight to see that these suppressed emotions can cause physical problems. We use tension, hyperventilation (over breathing), physical illness, addictions to alcohol, drugs, sleep, power, work, TV, sports, gambling, searching for relationships, money, even compulsive talking and use of the telephone—any number of mechanisms—to contain the fear and emptiness of our "inner child." This is how we build up a wall of neurosis (see my book *Anxiety & Depression: A Natural Approach*), which can lead to physical illness.

"Neurosis" should not be used as a disparaging word to describe what we consider odd behavior in someone else; it simply means a reaction to trapped pain. It is an "inner child," and consequently a soul (or whatever you will call your higher self) longing to be acknowledged, loved, and brought together to make a whole person—a person who is centered, peaceful within oneself, one's creator, and the world.

PART II

By Karen Brody

Guidelines for a Strict Candida Diet

Imagine that your body is a car. When a car is full of the right fuel it runs smoothly. If you put regular gasoline into a car that only runs on premium the car will become sluggish and perform poorly. The same is true about your body. If you put the right food in, you run smoothly. The wrong food can cause havoc.

A person with candida fits perfectly into this analogy. When you eat certain foods that the candida likes to "feed" on—bread, sugar, and mushrooms—your body will feel sluggish and a multitude of unpleasant symptoms can occur. These foods are the wrong fuel for your body. By eating a diet of foods that do not "feed" candida—one that includes fresh vegetables and grains—the candida has nothing to "feed" on and you soon gain the potential to feel better. These foods are the right fuel for your body.

As you read through this book, you will discover that food is a very powerful tool for healing yourself. You eat food every day, yet you rarely stop, look, and listen to what food is doing to your body. Ignoring the crucial role food plays in maintaining good health may have led to your current physical dis-ease. I intentionally hyphenate the word "dis-ease" to remind you that contracting a disease is your body's way of saying it is no longer "at ease." With the right food in your body, combined with other therapeutic approaches, your body can regain the strength to feel "at ease" again.

My Story

A number of years ago—after going to countless doctors for migraines, panic attacks, tingling in my shoulder, hands, and feet—I ended up at the office of a chiropractor and kinesiologist named Heidi. I almost canceled the appointment that day because I was skeptical that anything not involving a medical prescription would work, and because I was afraid of the physical act of getting to her office.

At the last moment I jumped into a taxi and went. I felt so low and had lost hope, assuming after going from doctor to doctor that my multisymptomatic problems meant I either had a terminal illness or I was crazy. My initial visit with Heidi lasted two hours. I almost threw up on her twice. Naturally I assumed the worst.

"You have something called candida," she said with confidence. "It's an overgrowth of yeast in your body."

"Why has this happened?" I asked.

"There are many reasons. The fact that you have been on antibiotics continually for a year and a half is one good reason."

"So what do I do?" I said, expecting to be given another prescription.

"Go home and have some carrot juice, eat millet, and wear orange. We'll talk about your new dietary requirements tomorrow."

I left her office thinking she was a freak. Have some carrot juice, eat millet, and wear orange? What kind of a treatment was that? How could food make me feel better? I had been in a health food store before but it always felt like I was a visitor rather than going in there with the intention of buying something. Confused about her diagnosis and method of treatment, but feeling so awful I would try anything that night, I bought millet and carrot juice at a health food store and dug out the only piece of orange clothing I owned. To my surprise, my body felt calmer than it had in months.

The next day she gave me a list of foods I should and should not eat to help the candida clear up. I was in shock—everything I was currently eating I was to stop eating. My life felt like it had been flipped upside down. "I'm sorry," I barked at Heidi, "but I don't cook; I don't have any time to cook; and I definitely do not know how to cook these strange foods."

With a smile on her face she said, "Go buy yourself a cookbook. Any cookbook that feels right for you."

I did and it changed my life.

I must admit, however, that I never would have found the motivation to change my diet if I had not felt so ill. To feel bad every day and have a number of doctors tell you they do not know why you feel that way feels like a punishment. At night I even cried out, "I want to die! Please let me die!" So when Heidi told me to change my diet and I would feel better, I thought what do I have to lose? Nothing, really.

While talking to many candida sufferers while researching this book I discovered my experience was not uncommon. Many people recounted horror stories about endless visits to their unsympathetic doctor, bathroom cabinets full of prescription drugs, panic attacks while driving, not wanting to get out of bed in the morning, or feeling like death was just around the corner. Their road to good health sometimes came only after much trial and error.

Changing to a New Healthier Diet

This section of *Candida: A Natural Approach* will tell you what to eat when you have a severe case of candida, but this is only one step in your new dietary regimen. You also have to know how to cope on a candida diet. How do you introduce new foods into your diet like soy milk and rice cakes while giving up foods like cookies and coffee? Where is yeast hiding in some of the most common foods you eat? How can you get your family and friends to try the same foods you eat?

There are many strict "dos" and "don'ts" on a diet to starve the candida that is thriving in your system, but following these rules doesn't have to be the worst experience of your life. As nutritionist Penny Davenport told me, "The good news is a candida diet is actually very healthy; if people stick to it they *will* feel better."

It's true, you will feel better on this diet. Once the yeast begins to die —for some that will take a few months, for others it will take longer— your life will change. Countless numbers of former candida sufferers have said, "It is like a cloud lifting from your head."

Candida specialists stress that if you do not change your diet you will not get rid of severe candida. You can take antifungals, probiotics, vitamins, and try many other natural remedies, but none of these alone will get you better—you also need to change your diet.

Is a Candida Diet Different for Women, Men, or Children?

The key to being on a successful candida diet—no matter what your age or sex—is to design your own personal daily regimen, bearing in mind the candida diet guidelines provided in this book *and* your personal needs. For example, most men need more to eat for lunch than a salad. Some experts also suggest that men eat more animal protein foods, while women should eat more vegetables. Diet expert Annemarie Colbin says this is perhaps because men discharge protein, carbohydrates, and minerals faster than women.

Everyone has a different body with different needs. The food one person can eat may not be what another person can tolerate. Likewise, the amount of food one person eats may not be the right amount for another. Honor your unique eating needs and use this book as a guideline. Good health is just around the corner.

CHAPTER NINE

What Foods You Need to Heal

The Limits of Modern Medicine

Your health is in your own hands. Modern medicine can be useful to some extent but it has limits. Consider this scenario. Jane goes to her doctor because she has been getting headaches. Her doctor prescribes a drug that gets rid of the headache but causes nausea. She then takes another drug to counterattack the nausea, but that irritates her stomach. For one year Jane lives on antacid pills to relieve her stomachache. Eventually she goes back to her doctor who refers her to a consultant who finds that she has developed an ulcer, for which he prescribes medication. Jane continues to eat the same diet she has always been on, foods loaded with sugar and lots of dairy products. The medication relieves some of her discomfort but she still finds she has to rely on antacids. One year later, still complaining of a "funny tummy" to her doctor, it is suggested she might be suffering from anxiety and might want a drug to relieve the anxiety.

Jane's health is out of control. Neither she nor her doctor is in control of it any more. She is not getting better and, at best, will continue to feel bad unless she takes control. Many people who have candida will be very familiar with Jane's scenario. Remember, you *can* take control of your health.

Annemarie Colbin, author of *Food and Healing*, sees three major errors in the assumptions we make about health and illness today. They are

- the belief that our physical symptoms (headaches, pimples, fevers) are erroneous reactions of the body to normal stimuli

- the belief that having surgery or taking a chemical substance, whether of natural or artificial origin, can restore health by interrupting the process called "disease"

- the belief that dietary habits are unrelated to symptoms or illness

All three of these assumptions are important to consider when you are trying to restore your health. You must get to know your body, listen to the subtle indications it gives you that add up to that I-don't-feel-well feeling and learn what unique methods your body needs in order to heal itself. A doctor cannot do the work you need to do in order for you to become healthy.

The Importance of Food in Healing

The body hates imbalance. When you cut yourself your body quickly restores its balance by forming a scab, which eventually falls off, and the skin returns to normal. In a similar way, eating "good" food will create a feeling of balance, allowing the immune system to spend its time healing. Too much "bad" food will throw the body off-balance, halting its natural instinct to heal. When you lack balance in your life —whether it is physical, emotional, or mental—you often feel bad physically. A good diet is one crucial step toward making you feeling better.

Many people have studied the effects of food and its ability to make us feel good and bad. In Kristina Turner's *Self-healing Cookbook* she makes it clear that foods and moods are directly related. She believes that certain foods nurture different organs, producing different effects in the body. For example, eating grains such as rye, barley, wheat, and quinoa helps cleanse the liver and gallbladder, producing a patient, flexible feeling in your mood. Some foods are more likely to cause disease, like dairy products, which have been linked to many female gynecological problems. In moderation, any food may be okay, but studies show that our contemporary society doesn't eat in moderation any more. If you combine our poor diets with the amount of chemicals going into the air, food, and water, it is not surprising that immunological diseases such as cancer and asthma are rampant today.

If you have candida your body is out of balance. The key is to bring it back into balance. Thinking about what you eat, how it will make you feel, and what it will do to your body will help to restore your body into the healthy state it wants to be in.

Foods Candida Sufferers Should and Should Not Eat

The biggest complaint I have heard from people with candida is that each book on candida suggests something different to eat. One says "yes" you can eat some sugars like fruit, and others say absolutely "no" to fruit. Obviously this is very confusing. My best advice is to choose one candida diet and stick with it. Do not overwhelm yourself with the contradictions you see in different diets. These contradictions exist mainly because, like any disease, what is right for you will be different than what is right for another. Everyone has different bodies and different degrees of candida. If your friend, who also has candida, can eat one piece of fruit every week but you can't, remember we are all different.

Foods to Avoid

Candida likes to "feed" on sweet and fermented or yeast-containing foods—often the foods you crave if you have candida. When you begin a candida diet most experts advise that you avoid a large number of the foods that feed the candida for at least three to four months. Depending on the severity of your condition, after a given time period you might be able to ease up a bit. Remember, especially in the beginning, if you follow the diet only 75 percent of the time you will still be feeding the candida. Natural supplements used to kill the yeast will help but they cannot do *all* the work in your body. You need to clean up your immune system by not eating foods that make you feel bad. Colbin points out, "Often it is not just what you eat, but also what you don't eat that helps you become healthy again."

The major foods you must avoid are

- foods containing yeast—bread, pizza

- foods containing sugar—most common breakfast cereals, puddings, honey, syrups, chocolate, cookies, canned drinks, most canned vegetables, products with malt, and endless others

- foods containing cow's milk, including cheese and cream

- fermented foods and drinks—alcohol, foods containing vinegar (ketchup, pickles, baked beans), soy sauce

- foods containing fungi and mold—mushrooms, nuts that are not fresh (nuts still in their shell are best), and leftover food (mold can grow on food overnight!)

- refined carbohydrates—white flour, white rice, white floured pasta, and anything not made from whole grains

- stimulants—colas, coffee, and tea, even decaffeinated

- smoked or cured foods—smoked or cured fish, ham, bacon, and any other cured meat.

Looking at the list above you must now be thinking, "So what can I eat?" The list is just as long.

Foods You Can Eat

The major foods you can eat are

- yeast-free breads—soda bread, chapatis (Indian flat bread), tortillas

- meat, poultry, and fish—it is best to buy organic, though, because most meat today contains antibiotics and hormones that are not good for anyone with an already weak immune system (especially women—eating meat or fish that contains hormones can contribute to dramatic hormonal swings in your body). If you cannot buy organic meat, non-organic lamb and rabbit are safer meats to eat because they are not mass produced and are less likely to be given hormones and antibiotics.

- potatoes—they can be a lifesaver when you go out to eat but remember if you get a baked potato ask them to stuff it with something that will not feed the candida—don't smother it with chili or cheese!

- grains—those that have been processed the least are best. Unfortunately, it would be best to avoid wheat, especially when you are just starting your diet because it has often been through a lot of processing and often contains mold. However, there are other grains such as millet, brown rice, quinoa, spelt, and amaranth, that you can eat instead.

- beans and legumes—great for so many meals—stews, casseroles, even burgers (freshly cooked beans, soaked overnight, are best to eat, but canned beans without added sugar are fine if you are in a hurry)

- unhydrogenated margarines—any dairy-free, unhydrogenated ones

- rice cakes flat breads—make great snacks, just read the ingredients before you buy them so you know exactly what you're eating

- fresh vegetables—your body needs fresh vegetables for their nutrients, so steam them, make a soup or stew, and discover all the many ways there are to enjoy fresh vegetables. Avoid canned vegetables because they usually come with sugar and preservatives. Get into the habit of buying your vegetables fresh, organic if you can, and eating salads daily.

- herbal tea, mineral water, and vegetable juice—discover the joy of juicing vegetables because it's a good way to get lots of nutrients into your diet. Try hot water on its own or with a bit of lemon—remember, your body needs water (not just any liquid, it should be water) to aid in the release of toxins, so drink six to eight glasses of filtered water per day.

- flours—any flour but white, processed flours are okay, but try to stay away from wheat at the beginning of your diet because of the mold. Experiment with other grain-based flours such as brown rice, soy, or millet flour (if you want to eat pasta look for pasta made with wheat-free flour)

- alternatives to cow's milk—soy milk, oat milk, rice milk, and nut milks are very nice. Or try goat, sheep, or soy cheese

- foods that have antifungal effects—garlic, leeks, chives, and onions are all wonderful foods to eat in abundance on a candida diet because they kill off fungi, molds, and viruses, but not friendly bacteria (you can prevent the smell of garlic on your breath by eating sprigs of fresh parsley with the garlic)

Beginning to add these foods into your diet might seem overwhelming at first. "How am I ever going to substitute soy milk for cow's milk, herbal tea, or, even worse, hot water for coffee?" Chapters Ten and Eleven will introduce you to some of these new foods and offer hints on how to make the transition to this new diet. Don't worry, many people have done it!

The Problem with Sugar

Sugar. We love it. Many of us think we can't live without it. Well, you have to. Candida loves sugar—it could eat sugar all day and night. Most likely, candida and the sugar you eat have been having a party in your system for a long time. When you stop eating sugar the party will end.

Here are some facts about sugar. The word "sugar" has two meanings. The first is the more popular definition of sugar, the sweet crystalline or powdered substance, spooned into coffee or used to make cookies and cakes. The second meaning is chemical: the sweet tasting, crystalline carbohydrates that are part of many foods you eat like maltose (sugar derived from malted grain), fructose (from fruit), and lactose (from milk). Usually any ingredient ending in "tose" means it is a form of sugar. This is important to remember when you are shopping. You must read the ingredients of everything you buy because sugar hides everywhere.

Sugar depresses the immune system. When you eat sugar it goes into your body and begins to metabolize. To do this it must take what nutrients it is missing from other sources in your body. This means taking from your reserve of nutrients—mostly B vitamins, calcium, phosphorus, and iron.

Everybody has a different limit to how many nutrients can be depleted from their body before they become nutritionally deficient and sick, but you can be sure that if you eat a lot of sugar your immune system has to work harder to stay healthy. You can also be sure that the candida in your body is feeding off this sugar and multiplying, making you feel rotten. Every person's body is different so it is pointless to try and figure out how much sugar it will take before you, your family, or your friends get to the point of feeling bad. It is better to eliminate sugar from your diet and eliminate candida's food source.

The Problems with Dairy Products

I used to be an ice cream addict. A tub of Häagen Dazs, a large spoon and some evenings that would be my supper. I never thought I could give it up, never, but I managed to make it through a year dairy-free. To reward myself I ate a tub of Häagen Dazs coffee ice cream. I felt human again (not to mention a little sick). The second year seemed less difficult, mainly because my body now felt stronger than it had in previous years and the multitude of health problems that had plagued me had virtually disappeared. Could dairy products have been a major culprit?

You probably have been brought up to believe that eating a lot of dairy products is good for you, will give you strong bones, and is just plain healthy. For most people, and candida sufferers in particular, too many dairy products are making our bodies feel sluggish and our immune systems weak. How?

Imagine a meal of cheese, a cream sauce, and ice cream going through the digestive process in your body. All of these are thick and dense. When they meet the various organs in the digestive system in large quantities they have a hard time getting through, and, like a sieve after you have pressed fruit through it, the pores get clogged. If you eat a lot of dairy products on a daily basis your organs cannot handle the overload; the excretion processes will not function properly. The result may be that you excrete the excess waste from other areas of your body, like your skin (you may have acne), or it stays in your body, building up and often forming mucus or pus, which is a perfect medium for bacteria to grow. Candida thrives on undigested milk for just this reason: the moldy, bacteria-filled environment of the mucus is a comfortable place for it to grow.

Dairy products also produce the perfect environment for other infections to develop. Many common health problems today have to do with the body trying to cope with the build-up and excretion of toxins in the body: asthma, allergies, acne, pimples, obesity, to name just a few. Dairy products are certainly not always the cause of excess build-up of toxins, but they are a contributing factor and must be considered if someone eats a lot of dairy products and is frequently experiencing ill health.

Women tend to suffer more from the build-up of dairy products than men, and it takes longer for them to get such build-ups out of their systems. Some researchers believe there is a link between the high consumption of dairy products by women and diseases like breast cancer and gynecological problems. I know when I cut out dairy products, the cysts on my ovaries that I had suffered from chronically for years disappeared and my periods were regular for the first time in my life. Many allergy specialists now tell people who consume a lot of dairy products and are sick all the time to cut them out of their diet and see how they feel. Often the difference is remarkable.

On the candida diet you can eat goat's and sheep's milk, but not cow's milk. This is because cow's milk is the most difficult to digest. It is mass produced and, as a result, often contains drug residues that an already sluggish body does not need in its system.

Allergies and Food Intolerance

For candida sufferers, knowing exactly what to eat is often complicated by allergies and food intolerance. You must be aware of these because you could change to a candida diet and still feel bad. Almost every person with candida suffers from an allergy or intolerance of at least one food; often they are allergic to many. This is because the candida weakens the immune system. You may get a headache, stomachache, a rash—allergic reactions come in many forms. An allergic reaction is your body's way of telling you, "No, I don't want this (food, environment) right now."

How You Tell an Allergy from an Intolerance

It is generally agreed by traditional allergists and other practitioners who test for allergies that an allergy is the immune system's response to a foreign substance. If you are allergic to a particular food the body's immune system will go on alert, produce antibodies, and an adverse reaction will occur.

This is about all that the medical establishment and other allergy practitioners agree on. Views on allergies are wide ranging, some specialists claiming that allergies do not cause severe medical problems while others insist that allergies are often the culprit behind many of the common health problems that exist today. Candida experts agree with the latter view and feel that you must identify what foods you are allergic to before you begin the candida diet. If not, you could be setting yourself up for disappointment because you will still be eating the wrong foods for you.

A food intolerance is similar to an allergy in that it is a reaction someone has to a foreign substance. Intolerance, or "sensitivities" as some allergists refer to them, are not recognized as readily by the traditional medical establishment as are allergies because they cannot be measured in a scientific way. Despite this, many natural health practitioners are convinced that food intolerances exist in people whose immune systems are weak. Factors like candida, stress, PMS, and digestive problems can cause intolerance to flare, and then you may only need a small amount of a food to cause a reaction.

In the book *Food Allergies* by Liz Earle (1995), the differences between an allergy and an intolerance are summed up in the following way: "True food allergies are easier to detect because there is a reaction every time that food is eaten. Food intolerances are like shifting sands in the sense that the body may or may not react every time, depending on what else is going on. However, the symptoms are much the same for both and can affect almost any part of the body."

How to Know What Foods You Are Allergic To

When you begin your treatment for candida it is best to see an allergist to help identify which foods you react to. The most common food sensitivities are to:

- wheat
- dairy products
- yeast
- corn
- eggs
- beef
- citrus fruits

Until you begin to know your body better and go to a practitioner to identify your allergies there are some self-tests you can do at home.

Start a Food Diary

This can give you a good idea of what foods you are putting into your body and how they make you feel. Write down everything you eat for one week and the time you eat it. Also write down any physical symptoms you feel and the day and time they occur. At the end of the week look back at your diary to see if there is any correlation between the food you ate and how you felt. If you suspect one or more foods are giving you problems eliminate them and see how you feel.

One of the major drawbacks of this test is that often, if you eat out, you do not know what ingredients are in your food so it may be difficult to identify your problem foods. Also, sometimes you may have delayed reactions to foods—the reaction occurring several days later.

You need to be aware of these drawbacks but don't let them prevent you from trying this test—many people do identify food allergies this way.

Elimination Diet

For one week do not eat all the common foods to which you think you are sensitive. If your symptoms subside, continue on the diet for one more week, then begin to add back the eliminated foods, only one per day. Be careful not to add an eliminated food in a form that contains another one of your eliminated foods. For example, if you are eliminating wheat and eggs, don't eat something with wheat that also contains eggs because then you cannot be sure which one you are reacting to. If symptoms do occur after you have reintroduced a food you probably should avoid that food for a while. To be sure, recheck the food by eating it at five-day intervals to make sure it was not a coincidence that you developed symptoms after eating it.

If your symptoms are not alleviated at all by an elimination diet then it is possible you are not allergic to the foods you eliminated and you should consider eliminating other foods or look at environmental factors in your life, such as dust or household chemicals, which commonly cause problems for candida sufferers.

The elimination diet can be done by yourself, but people who know they have serious allergic reactions, like asthmatics and small children, are advised to test foods in this way under the supervision of an allergy specialist.

Avoid drugs. Try not to treat a food intolerance with drugs without first trying to cure it by eliminating different foods. (Of course, an allergic reaction to a food—to peanuts, for example—needs immediate treatment.) It makes no sense, especially if you have candida, to use drugs because they can also feed the candida. In addition, they only treat the symptoms, not the cause of your reaction. If you want to treat the cause, identify which foods produce your ill feelings and eliminate those foods from your diet. Most people feel remarkably better when they do this.

DETOXING

When you eliminate certain foods from your diet your body will experience a "die-off" reaction because the candida has nothing to feed on any more. Also, because the foods you are allergic to have built up in your system and they are no longer entering it, they begin to break down and find their way out of the body. Initially you may feel worse before you feel better, but do not be scared or put off by an increase in symptoms because it means that your body is getting rid of all the substances that have been causing the problems. Indeed, Michio Kushi, a leader of the macrobiotic movement (dedicated to healthy, spiritual, and vegan living), describes detoxing as the body's way of "house cleaning." He says any of the following symptoms can be experienced when your body detoxes:

- general fatigue
- pains and aches
- fever, chills, coughs
- abnormal sweating and frequent urination
- skin discharges and unusual body odors
- diarrhea and constipation
- temporary decrease in sexual vitality and desire
- temporary cessation of menstruation
- irritability
- minor transitory symptoms, such as a little hair loss, restless dreams, feeling cold

Only some of these symptoms will be experienced by most people who are detoxing, depending on how bad your candida and food allergies are. The more your body has to clean out, though, the stronger and longer the reaction will be to your body's cleansing process. Everyone detoxes at different rates so comparing yours with another person's is pointless.

Do not discontinue your diet because of detoxification symptoms (see the "Food Elimination and Symptom Chart" on page 181).

Friends and family may say, "Why are you on that diet if it makes you so sick?" Tell them you're on it because you are actually getting better! Once you go through the detoxification period most people do feel a lot better. It's like coming out of a dark tunnel into sunlight.

Listening to Your Inner Guide to Know What to Eat

We all know what we should eat yet rarely do we listen to our bodies. Having regular "conversations" with your body is an excellent way to be able to gauge what food is right for you. This may initially sound silly.

Colbin suggests doing the following. Relax for a few minutes with your eyes closed. Send a message down to your body just like you were beaming a sonic wave to the bottom of the ocean. Ask yourself, "Is this (pick a food) good for me?" A distinct feeling will well up. "Yes," it's okay, or "no," it's wrong. Go with your gut feeling.

Colbin stresses one crucial thing to keep in mind while doing this exercise. "Okay" feelings about food are not to be confused with "delicious." Ice cream may be "delicious," but it will not evoke an "okay" feeling. Don't forget this advice when you practice this exercise.

Our bodies are constantly giving us "yes/no" signals, telling us what we really want to eat. As you become more in tune with your body you should instinctively know when to reintroduce foods into your diet.

Case Histories

The stories that follow take you through some of the highs and lows you could expect when you go on a strict candida diet. As you read them remember that everyone's body has different needs. What is the right road to recovery for one person may not be the right road for you. Even if what works for you is different from what works for other candida sufferers, the stories in this chapter show that you are not alone in your quest to regain your health by changing your diet. Many people have done this and succeeded in ridding their bodies of candida.

MY FAMILY THOUGHT I WAS CRAZY

Sarah had rheumatoid arthritis for years and decided to get help because she did not want to continue taking medication to control her arthritis forever. She saw a friend get a lot better after cutting out foods from her diet so she decided to go to that friend's health practitioner. When Sarah was told she had candida she was flabbergasted.

To be honest, I didn't really think food was as important as I do now. I mean, you eat things and sometimes after you might think, "Oh, I didn't like that" or "I feel a bit sick," but I still used to eat them. It never registered, don't eat these things.

When I was handed the sheet of paper telling me what to eat on this candida diet it was frightening. I thought, "I'm not going to be able to eat anything." And things I liked I could not eat. I always used to love coffee. In the morning a cup of coffee—oh!—I wouldn't dream of getting up and doing anything without a cup of coffee. When I saw "no coffee" on the diet I thought, "I'm not going to be able to do this. It can't be right, people have drunk coffee for years." I did do it, but it was very, very hard. But I thought I wasn't going to lose anything by giving it a chance.

Having a family made it difficult because you've still got to buy things that you can't have, but they can. Like gravy. I used to love gravy. I hated a dinner if there wasn't a nice gravy. A lovely gravy finishes the dinner—so that was hard when you're having your dinner dry. Sometimes I poured cauliflower or cabbage water over the dinner, but I like my meal to look colorful and it looked awful. The taste wasn't too bad though. All along I was telling myself, "It's nice, I am going to like this," because I didn't want to ache. And now I don't even think of having gravy.

My family all thought I was crazy. They would say to me "What are you doing that for? Why don't you eat this?" I got no support whatsoever. I sometimes thought at first I was crazy. For years and years people have had these foods and then someone all of a sudden is telling you not to eat them.

If I cheated—and many times in the beginning I did cheat— my kids used to say, "Oh, you're having a cookie! You can't do that!" And I think they got pleasure out of saying that. It is hard, and after a while you think, "Oh, I must be all right now. I could just have that cookie." Especially when I have my period my taste buds go crazy and sometimes I'm thinking, "No, don't do it!" The next thing I'd be opening the cupboard again thinking, "What are you doing?" Everybody's different with cheating. One of my friends with candida is great. She is a saint. But me, I found it hard not to cheat, especially at first.

When I'd go to my Mother's house I used to take all my own food with me and not eat her food. My Mother thought I was crazy as well. My family's reaction was, "Oh, we don't think it'll do you any harm. I've been eating that for years and there's nothing wrong with me." You get to the point after a while where you tend to keep quiet about it with certain people. But my friends were great about my new diet. At Christmas or at parties they'd just fix me a baked potato in the oven. It was fine and they were really good about it.

At work I used to take food with me. The diet is really just about altering your patterns a bit and preparing something to take with you. Usually I'd just get something at work—a sandwich or something—but now I have to give myself time to prepare something. Once I've done it, it's nothing really. Just altering my patterns. The same with food shopping. I have to look to see what's in things. Like tomatoes, I'm allergic to tomatoes. There are so many things with tomatoes in them. In the beginning you think there is nothing you can eat, but it's amazing how you find alternatives.

Going out was difficult because you don't always know all the ingredients in the meal. Now I do go out but I choose something plain that I know I can eat. Baked potatoes are my favorite.

When you start the diet it's like going into a jungle and you don't ever think you're going to get out. After six months I did start to feel a lot better. And now it's become a way of life for me. I feel I've got energy in me. Before I used to just trudge on, now I can jump, unless I start eating a lot of cookies and candy. I feel good all the time—and I'm off my arthritis medication!

I WAS ALLERGIC TO EVERYTHING

Nine years ago, 43-year-old Louise, despite eating huge amounts of food, was so thin her doctor decided it was due to her gallbladder so he had it removed. A few months later, still unusually thin, her doctor was not able to explain what was wrong with her. Then a friend of a friend recommended that she see a clinical ecologist. Willing to do anything, Louise went to see him.

He immediately tested me for food allergies and I was allergic to all citrus fruits, dairy products, sugar, and chocolate. It was funny because I had already cut out tea and coffee because I knew they were bad for me. Instead, I was drinking only citrus juice. No wonder I was feeling so bad!

Initially he did not know I had candida, but he told me to eliminate the foods I had tested allergic to. I did and felt better for the first five days. But then the malaise came back across my eyes and all I wanted to do was put my head down. For six weeks it continued and I felt like I was going crazy. I would walk down the supermarket aisle and want to buy anything that had sugar in it.

I went back to him and this time he tested to see if I had candida. Well, I did. Back then not much was known about candida, but he did give me a diet sheet so I knew what I could and could not eat.

The diet was very difficult at first, but I was so sick I wanted to try anything. I never cheated—it just wasn't worth it to me. But when you are sick you lose your confidence so I became a totally different person at work. People thought I was a very withdrawn person when, in fact, just the opposite had been true!

My husband was a tower of strength. He ate a lot of my new foods with me (but would still have his desserts). This was crucial in my recovery. I was living on only about five foods in my diet for many years because it ended up I was allergic to everything. All flours, all cooked root vegetables, all nuts and seeds. . . . There was practically nothing I could snack on but I felt so much better when I did not eat these foods that it was worth it.

I now laugh at how uncomfortable it makes people feel when I go for tea and order hot water. The other day this happened with my Mother. When I first started on this diet I had a difficult time asking for hot water. I always offered to pay for it, not wanting them to think I was poor and trying to get a hand-out. But now I've realized that if I want hot water it's okay. So I just order it.

How has being on a candida diet changed my life? Well, next week my husband and I are off to Portugal for a vacation. Nine years ago I rarely left my house. I also never have to go to doctors because I never get sick much. And my weight is finally normal.

I WANTED TO EAT WHAT EVERYBODY ELSE ATE

Throughout childhood Phil was always getting sick with colds and sinus infections. By his teenage years he was taking antibiotics regularly. His tonsils were removed when he was 15, which provided some relief, but at 19 he began to work in a factory and experienced severe headaches, fatigue, and Irritable Bowel Syndrome. His doctor gave him medication and some dietary advice, but nothing seemed to work.

I was feeling worse and worse. Every day just to get out of bed was difficult—an effort. I didn't know what to do any more. My doctor didn't know what to do with me. Luckily my wife's friend suggested I see her nutritionist.

She tested me for allergies. I was allergic to everything. Unbelievable, I thought. No way—can't be—but then after I got more information from the nutritionist I thought again and it did make sense. I must have had allergies my whole life.

When I was handed the candida diet sheet I thought it was ridiculous. How was I ever going to eat like that? Impossible. I went home and showed my wife the diet and she also thought it just wouldn't be possible. But then we decided if this diet was what it was going to take to make me feel better then I'd better give it a try.

Where I work everyone brings a packed lunch and we eat together. At lunchtime every day I ate a sandwich. Every day. Everyone eats a sandwich. Also, if you don't eat with people they'll start talking. I felt really foolish the first day I brought my lunch on the candida diet. My wife made me a baked potato and I took that and a can of tuna. When it was lunchtime I wanted to say I wasn't hungry, but everyone knows how much I usually eat so that wouldn't work. So I ate my tuna and potatoes. Everyone laughed at first. They laughed for a while. In the evening I'd go home and say to my wife, "I just want to eat what everyone else is eating." She was really helpful and gave me encouragement to continue—I wouldn't have been able to do it without her.

The other hard habit to change was going for a pint of beer after work or on the weekends. I loved having my beer. At first I couldn't face going to the bar with friends after work. I always said I was busy after work. Some people made a comment but I didn't care because I just couldn't face it. Now I do go and have no problem ordering a soda water. When I started feeling better from this diet I became less concerned about eating and drinking foods that were different from those of other people.

I can't believe how much energy I have now. And my relationship with my wife has improved a lot because when I felt bad all the time I couldn't be nice. I'm like a different person now and all because I was eating the wrong foods for my body before. Imagine that.

CHEATING IS A VICIOUS CYCLE

Six years ago Katie felt sluggish and always had pains in her knees and legs. She had taken the Pill for ten years and had experienced gynecological problems throughout her adult years. She remembers as a child she was always fussy about food. She used to take notes to school that said, "Katie does not like this. Don't give her this in her school meal."

I've always had an open mind and believed that a lot of the illnesses are from the foods we eat. When I was given the candida diet sheet I thought, "I can't do it," but I'd paid the money to go and see this allergist so I thought I had to give it a shot.

I changed my diet the day after I saw the allergist. In the beginning I felt a bit tearful—I didn't understand I was going through withdrawal. I found with the least little thing I was crying; it was as if I had lost my confidence, which was not like me. My husband didn't understand it but was very easygoing about changing his diet. He said, "Well, that's fine by me. I'll have what you're having." Now we primarily eat what I call "wholesome" food.

It has not been easy sticking to the diet. Last week I had a couple of bad days because I cheated. I bought a muffin and I ate some chocolate and I felt terrible. I'm just starting to get back into the diet. I seem to go down at Christmas time—I have no willpower. I start eating a few sweets and then it's like a vicious cycle. It's easy to start feeling poorly again and then it's harder to get off those foods. And I know sometimes when I'm eating the foods that are bad for me that I'm going to be ill tomorrow, but I can't stop myself.

Last summer I went back to my allergist and I told him I did not feel good and that I had been cheating. He said, "Look, you're wasting your money coming here because you have got to do it yourself." So I went home and thought, "Well, yes, I am stupid." I had gone for a few months and didn't cheat, but chocolate is my most difficult challenge. And as soon as

Christmas comes, you know, you're bringing candy for other people and then you think, "I'll just have one. One won't hurt me." But, of course, one leads to two and so on.

When I was very strict on the diet I could get up and climb mountains. There's no doubt about it, the diet does work. Now I've cut out corn flakes because, funnily enough, since I was okay on soy milk I was also told I could have a few corn flakes. Well, I was eating four or five bowls a day and, in the end, when I got tested for allergies again I was sensitive.

My friends thought I'd gone a bit crazy when I first went on the diet. So did my sister, but she is always at the doctor— always. A week does not go by without her visiting the doctor. I've tried to tell her—she knows she's allergic to so many foods but she eats everything. Her food is her comfort in life. I think for many of us it is that way, but it has to change.

If I go out for a meal I will call the restaurant beforehand and order a separate meal. People at restaurants don't mind that, they are geared to it—especially with lots of vegetarians around now—and they are pretty good. At first I felt uncomfortable about asking for a special meal. We would go from one restaurant to the other. I'd look at the menu and say, "Oh no, I've got to leave here—there's nothing I can eat" and so rather than ask them to do something special I would just leave. Now I don't care; I just ask them.

I have had people over to eat and cooked my foods. When they ask "What's this?" I say it's ground beef and they don't know it's tofu. Then after they've eaten it I tell them it's tofu and they can't believe it didn't taste any different. If I make people a sandwich and they say they'd like butter I use soy margarine and they don't know the difference.

I am healthy. I haven't had to go to the doctor for years. I don't take medication. It is expensive trying to get better, taking all the supplements, but I decided to spend my money on getting better. "Quality of life"—that's how I look at it.

Hopefully these stories have motivated you to start your candida diet soon. You *can* feel better. Each story in this chapter demonstrates this. The next chapter will help you get started on your road to recovery.

CHAPTER TEN

Getting Started on Your Diet

When I was first diagnosed with candida I was convinced this new diet would never fit into my lifestyle. I was in shock. Luckily my kinesiologist told me to "Go buy a cookbook." This was just what I needed to do. If I was going to get better I had to get started on the diet.

You, too, have to get started on the diet. Let go of all the negative thoughts: "I can't cook," "I have no time to cook," or "There will be nothing to eat when I go out to a restaurant." If you continue to think this way you will not succeed on this diet. The people who have had the most success are the ones who began the diet thinking positively and were willing to experiment with new ideas. A positive attitude makes for a positive outcome.

Below are a few ways you can make a positive start to your candida diet:

- *Make a commitment.* The sooner you get on the diet the quicker you will recover. Many candida sufferers ask, "Will I ever be able to eat "normal" food again?" (Ironically most people who have been on a candida diet now think processed, sugary foods are abnormal!) This diet does not have to be a lifelong commitment, but it does have to be for as long as it takes until you to feel better.

- *Take a whole-food cooking class.*   This is an excellent way to feel more comfortable cooking your new foods. Ask around if anyone in your area cooks whole foods or put an ad in your local paper. You may be surprised to find that one of your neighbors is a whole-food cook or knows one! Ask your local hospital if they give a cooking class or series of classes on cooking for special diets.

- *Read, study, and ask questions about candida.*   Read books on topics related to healing and special diet cookbooks. Ask someone at your local health food store for a recommendation or if they know someone in the area who could teach you more. Remember a lot of health-orientated people walk into health food stores so yours could be filled with information—if you ask!

- *Start where you are.*   Only you know which factors make this diet easy or hard for you to stick to. Take into account what your lifestyle is like. Are you a single mother with small kids? A newly married couple with a hectic work and social life? All of these factors must be taken into consideration when you design your candida diet.

Four Steps to Creating a Meal Plan

Once you have made the commitment to change your food habits and try new things, creating a candida meal plan can be enjoyable. You may think "I don't need a meal plan. I'll just start." That is okay if that's what feels right for you, but many people find it helpful to have a plan for at least the first month of the diet. A plan relieves the panic you feel when you return home from a long day and cannot think of anything to eat. If you take 30 minutes at the beginning of the month to plan your meals you don't have to waste precious energy the rest of the month figuring out what to eat.

A meal plan does not mean you are locked into a routine. On the contrary, a meal plan assists you in breaking free from eating routines.

Below is a four-step process for creating a candida meal plan. It is easy to follow and can get you on your way to eating a candida diet.

To create your own meal plan you will need:

- A quiet, relaxing space where you can think without interruption for 30 minutes
- A pencil (with an eraser) and a colored pen
- Several large index cards
- A list of the candida diet guidelines (see Chapter Nine of this book)
- A list of the foods you are allergic to or suspect you may be allergic to

STEP 1: CONSIDER ALL YOUR LIFESTYLE FACTORS

Answer the following questions on one index card. Put the heading "Lifestyle Factors" at the top of the page.

- How often do I eat at home? At work? Go out to eat?
- How much time do I have to prepare meals?
- Would the people I live with be willing to go on this diet with me and provide support?
- What three things are causing me the most stress in my life at this moment?

STEP 2: PICK FOODS YOU WANT TO EAT

Look at the list of foods permitted on a candida diet (pages 92–94) and the list of your food allergies. Make a list of all the foods you want to eat that you are not allergic to. Also write down foods you may have never tasted but are willing to try.

Put the heading "Candida Foods" at the top of the page. Then with a colored pen, indicate next to the food if it is "G" for "Grain," "B" for "Beans," "V" for "Vegetable," or "M" for "Meat." If you are a vegetarian obviously exclude the meat. If you are a meat eater you might eat fewer beans. These are the staples in a candida diet. Don't worry right now about any foods that don't fit into these categories.

STEP 3: DECIDE WHICH FOODS YOU ARE GOING TO EAT AND WHEN

Now you are ready to make your personal candida meal plan. Read through all the instructions in this section before you begin. Then take out your "Lifestyle Factors" list and your "Candida Foods" list.

On your index cards make a weekly calendar, using one card for each week. The first date on the calendar is the day you decide to start. Leave enough space on each day to fit your staple foods: grains, beans, vegetables, and meats.

On each day write which grains, beans, vegetables, and meats you will eat. I suggest working with one category at a time for the whole month; decide all the days you will eat grains that month, then all the days you'll eat beans, and so on.

Return to your "Lifestyle Factors" list often to remind yourself of your limits so your plan will be realistic. For example, on the days you know you'll have little time to cook, decide to eat foods that will allow you to make a quick meal, like corn pasta (G) with steamed vegetables (V) and Lemon, Garlic, and Oil Dressing. On a day you will be eating out think of what foods from your list you may be able to get at a restaurant, like a baked potato. Going on a candida diet is about altering your patterns.

Always be aware of the importance of rotating your foods in order to decrease the chances of becoming sensitive to more foods, which can happen when you eat too much of one food. To do this, as you fill in foods throughout the month make sure you're eating them every fourth day, not every day. Again, working with one category at a time makes this easier. For example, if you plan to eat rice on Monday you can eat rice again Friday, then Tuesday, then Saturday. If the range of foods you have to choose from is very limited because of food allergies then try to leave a day or two between eating the same foods. You must break out of food ruts! You may be able to eat a particular food today, but if you eat it every day for many weeks, most candida sufferers find that after a while they cannot tolerate that food any more.

STEP 4: MENU PLAN FOR THE WEEK

Now that you've decided which staple foods you want to eat each week, spend 15 minutes planning how to put them into your meals.

Look at your staple foods for each day and prepare meals around those foods. Always include a snack for the day for a quick fix. And remember to look at your "Lifestyle Factors" sheet to remind you of your limits. If your staples were brown rice (G), carrots (V), kale (V), leeks (V), and organic chicken (M), your menu for that day might look like this:

- Breakfast: Puffed brown rice and soy milk.

- Lunch: Carrot soup with brown rice and toasted sesame seeds (if you're taking a lunch with you, pack some brown rice cakes and a spread like hummus instead of the cooked brown rice, and bring the soup with you if you have access to cooking facilities).

- Dinner: Lemon gingered chicken, brown rice, and steamed carrots, kale, and a creamy leek sauce.

- Snack: Toasted sunflower seeds.

Balance and flexibility are the key to successful meal planning. When you are planning, keep in mind your current state of health, the weather (plan warming foods, like stews, for winter and cooling foods like salads for summer), your individual tastes, and, of course, your lifestyle factors.

Helpful Hints for Preparing Meals

Keep Meals Simple

Preparing fewer foods and eating them in their most natural state is healthier and often more enjoyable than creating something elaborate. Putting various ingredients in sauces and other dishes increases the risk of your reacting to those ingredients and increases your time in the kitchen. *Less is best.*

Yeast Can Hide in Your Kitchen

Old vegetables often have mold on them, especially if they are organic, because they haven't been sprayed with chemicals to retain a fresh look. Refrigerating your vegetables can help them keep longer. Nuts, oils, and seeds should be refrigerated because they will get moldy. Wooden cutting boards also carry yeast so clean them thoroughly or use plastic cutting boards.

Leftover food gets moldy so it is best to avoid food that has been prepared 24 hours beforehand. Most candida sufferers can get away with preparing food the night before and then eating it for lunch the next day, but some cannot. If your condition is this severe, avoid leftovers for a while.

Make a Shopping List

When you are beginning a candida diet, many of the foods you are going to eat will be new to you. Shopping with a list ensures that you will not forget the foods you need to buy. Use your menu plan to make a shopping list so you know what staples to buy. For vegetables, be flexible. If the ones on your list are not in the store or are not fresh, don't buy them, pick a different vegetable.

Learn Cooking Tricks

Cooking tricks can save you a lot of time. Read different cookbooks or go to cooking classes. Here are a few helpful tricks I have learned.

- *Cleaning leeks with ease*   Leeks can trap dirt between their layers so cut the leek in half lengthwise. Hold each half under running water, separating the layers to let the water run through them. When the dirt is out, turn them cut side down to drain.

- *Taking the peel off garlic*   Peeling garlic can be quick and easy. Put the garlic on a chopping board. Take a wide-blade knife, put the garlic under the flat part of the knife and press hard. The garlic skin should loosen so much that it almost falls off.

- *Softening beans and avoiding gas*   Soak beans overnight, even small beans like lentils. Discard the soaking water and add fresh water. Cook them together with *kombu*, a sea vegetable you can buy in health food stores. You can take the *kombu* out when you've finished cooking or leave it in and eat it!

Prepare the Same Basic Foods for Everyone

If the people you eat with at home are not eating your foods, you can still prepare the basic foods you eat, take out a portion for yourself, then add extra spices, ingredients or sauces for the others. Don't make more work for yourself by trying to prepare completely different meals for you and your family.

Atmosphere Is Important

What makes a good meal is not just the food. Flowers, an attractive tablecloth on the dining table, candles, and a plate of colorful food are all satisfying ways to brighten the atmosphere and nourish yourself and everyone else at the table. These "finishing touches" take surprisingly little time to do and are worth it.

Digestion or Indigestion: How to Eat

People rush around every day and when they have a moment quickly cram food into their mouths. And if you're not eating as quickly as you can, then you may be eating in an anxious, emotional state. Sometimes you are conscious of how worked up you are when you eat, but often you are not. The result of eating in a hurried or emotional state is indigestion. Proper digestion usually will not occur in a stressed or unhappy person.

Deepak Chopra, spokesperson on the mind-body link, believes that proper digestion will not occur if you continue with self-destructive eating patterns. In *Creating Health*, Chopra suggests guidelines that allow your mind and body to join together and help you digest and assimilate food properly:

1. Pay attention to eating

2. Pause momentarily before eating and sit in silence—or say grace—so that the awareness begins the meal quietly

3. Eat when you are hungry, and do not eat when you are not hungry

4. Do not sit down to eat if you are upset—your body is better off without food until you feel better

5. Take time to eat, chewing well and slowly

6. Appreciate the company and compliment the cook (even if it's yourself)

7. Avoid eating in any company that makes you feel less than agreeable, but rather eat with congenial company, friends, and family, when you can

Write these guidelines down, maybe on an index card so you can carry it around with you or put it on your refrigerator in the kitchen; before you eat, think about them. Maybe adopting every one now is not possible for you. I know that number four, "Do not sit down to eat if you are upset" is a real challenge for candida sufferers because you're always upset if you're feeling sick all over! Introduce one at a time and then, when you're ready, introduce another one. Being conscious of how to eat well is one of the quickest ways to good health. And as your mind gets better so will your digestion.

The Well-Stocked Kitchen

Having the right equipment in your kitchen is essential for a candida diet because you will be preparing fresh food on a daily basis. If you don't have the proper tools to make many of these dishes then it will be a lot more difficult to prepare the food you need for good health.

Every candida kitchen should have the following:

- *Food processor*   This relatively small financial investment will significantly increase your meal repertoire. Soups, hot cereals, spreads, and many more dishes become easy when you have a food processor.

- *Stainless steel or enamel cookware*   The pots and pans you use are important because whatever they are made of will get into your food and if the cookware is of poor quality you could feel sick. Do not use aluminum cookware because aluminum is a dangerous chemical. Studies have shown that when water is heated in an aluminum pot the aluminum level in the water increases by 75 percent. Most tap water is safer than this level. Stainless steel and enamel cookware, however, are safe and worth buying.

- *Good, sharp knives* Chopping vegetables with bad knives or unsharpened knives is a great way to frustrate yourself. Buy one large and one small knife of good quality and you'll feel born again. Keep them sharp and you will be able to happily chop away.

- *Plastic air-tight containers and glass jars* Containers and jars of different sizes, good quality, and with tight seals are crucial. You will have so many things to store—grains, leftovers for a day, food you want to freeze. Containers are also excellent for people on the go, for packing a lunch, or a snack. Jars are great for storing grains and legumes.

- *Resealable bags* You will use a lot of these if you work outside the home. They are also perfect for snacks and storing food.

- *Brush to clean vegetables* A good brush can make cleaning vegetables practically effortless. I have found that thick-bristled brushes work best.

- *Stainless steel steamer* An indispensable, cheap addition to your kitchen. These steamers fit in almost all pots and encourage you to get out of the habit of boiling your vegetables.

Think of buying

- *A juicer* Fresh vegetable juices taste wonderful and are full of nutrients.

- *Ginger grater* A grater makes using ginger easy—you don't need to chop the ginger up finely, just take off the skin and grate. Ginger is a miracle spice. It helps nausea and is heat-producing, so most candida sufferers should use a lot of it.

Every candida kitchen should *never* have the following:

- *Microwave* Sorry. I know most people have microwaves these days, but microwaves change the basic energy in food. Food that is microwaved will have little or no nutritional value. No definitive studies have been able to prove microwaves change the molecular structure of foods in a bad way, but most food experts agree that microwaving food makes the food less nutritious. This includes defrosting or reheating food in the microwave. The only exception I would make is (if you are not very sick) to allow yourself to use a microwave once in a while when you take food to work. Here a microwave might be the only way to reheat your food. For some candida sufferers who are very sensitive to their environment, however, just having a microwave in the kitchen that other people use could cause them to feel sick. If you must have a microwave for other people to use put it in a room you do not use very much.

How to Have Fun with Your New Foods

Have a Candida Dinner Party

Imagine your family or friends' responses to being served some of the foods on your candida diet. The more unusual the food, the funnier the response. You may think it's a bold move to have a candida dinner party but introducing your new foods to friends and family by allowing them to try them is usually a great way to make everyone more comfortable about your new diet. People may laugh at the food, but they are usually laughing only because they don't understand this way of eating. Demystify healthy eating for them.

Before the meal, learn a few interesting bits of information about the food you're serving, like the nutritional benefits of sea vegetables. Write this information in different colors on index cards and put the cards on the table before the meal. During the meal use these cards to explain the foods that are being served and why you need to eat them. Share your mixed feelings about cooking these foods and how you first felt making a dish with a new food. Invite your dinner guests to share their mixed feelings about eating this food. Allow the conversation to go anywhere. Usually, though, everyone will be *too* eager to express their feelings!

You may feel embarrassed and alone at first, but usually by the end of the meal you will feel more dedicated to your healing journey and very proud of yourself for taking a risk. Some recipe suggestions for a candida dinner party are found on page 175.

Theme Meals

This is a great way to get kids or your partner to try eating the candida diet foods. The foods may initially seem boring and tasteless, but with a little atmosphere and certain food combinations, you can have a meal everyone wants to eat.

Dress up in colorful garb, put candles on the table, play some Spanish music, and you have Mexican night. Or put on your blue jeans and a baseball cap, rent a baseball video, and you have "Yankee (or Dodger) Night." Put a blanket on the floor, eat with plastic cutlery and you have "Picnic Night." Any theme you choose is the right theme. Both kids and adults love it. See the menu suggestions on page 176 for the three themes mentioned here.

Find a Healing Friend

Finding someone you can relate to who also has candida or having a good friend who can empathize with you about your new foods and health needs is a crucial part of your recovery. Sometimes you just need to brainstorm with someone about how you're feeling and what you need to do about it. A good healing friend does this and also asks you for help. A good healing friend cooks with you and enjoys your cooking. A good healing friend makes you laugh, dance, or sing, and forget your troubles at just the right time. A good healing friend is that kindred spirit and a whole lot more.

If you cannot think of anyone who fits the "good healing friend" description then create your own. Sit quietly, close your eyes and imagine yourself walking through the woods. The path through the woods leads to a small cottage. At the door stands your healing friend. Now open your eyes and write that healing friend a letter; introduce yourself and tell her what you want in the friendship. Later on make a conscious effort to become this friend to people you meet and soon you will find a healing friend comes into your life. It could be a person you meet at a cooking class or an old friend. Enjoy her friendship and watch things change.

Eat from a Special Bowl or Plate

If you think your new foods are unexciting, spice them up with a special healing bowl or plate. A bright yellow bowl or a plate with lots of earth tones can be just the right addition that takes you out of the candida-diet blues. When I was feeling my worst with candida, my forest green Chinese-style bowl got me through a lot of sad moments. It represented stability and healing. I could always count on it to pick me up when I was feeling down. I also had an orange plate which symbolized the healing that needed to take place in my liver.

Learn which colors are said to heal various parts of your body and then buy a bowl in the color that heals the area that's out of balance. Alternatively, choose your favorite color. Buy any style and size of bowl or plate that is right for you. Chinese-style bowls are wonderful because you can eat any meal out of them.

Spend Time in a Health Food Store

This should be one of the first things you do when you start your diet. You may think, "They're so expensive," or "I don't know what to buy." Health food stores vary dramatically, but most have many affordable products (think of all the money you're saving not buying processed foods!). And there are lots of things you can buy in them that are yeast-free, dairy-free, and sugar-free. The sooner you get to your nearest health food store the better.

To make the most of your first trip, it is best to plan ahead. What products do you want to buy? If you have no idea, just remind yourself that whatever you buy it must be part of the candida diet so read the ingredients of every item. There are a lot of unhealthy foods even in health food stores. When you walk in, if you feel confident enough, ask to speak to someone who can help you identify foods suitable for a candida diet. (Bring your list of candida foods because some shopkeepers will not know.) This person may also be a good source of information about local cooking classes for special diets or new books on healing.

Once you begin to see the health food store as your friend in healing, eating candida foods will become easier.

Strategies for Eating Out

You *can* eat out. Of course every candida person is different and many stop going out for a while when they first go on the diet because eating out seems too difficult to cope with on top of all the other hurdles of the diet. If you want (or have) to go out to eat here are some strategies to ease the panic and make it enjoyable:

- Call the restaurant or host before you arrive and tell them your dietary needs. Most restaurants and all good hosts want to provide food you can eat. If you call the restaurant in the morning on the day you plan to go and ask to speak to the chef, she will most likely be happy to create a menu using foods you can eat. This was a difficult step for me to take, but the response I got was overwhelmingly positive. At a wedding I didn't tell the chef in advance about my dietary requirements so I expected to eat nothing. Once I said I needed special food, I was presented with a plate of vegetables and rice, the best meal I'd ever had at a wedding. Many people are getting used to catering to special diets, so don't feel shy—just ask!

- Find a favorite restaurant. Think about which restaurants there are in your area and find at least one that offers one or two dishes you can eat and enjoy. This is your safety restaurant. When friends or colleagues want to go out to eat suggest this restaurant.

- Eat something before you go. A snack or even a mini-dinner can be a lifesaver if you are going somewhere you think there might not be anything for you to eat. It is better to have something in your stomach than to sit at the table with an empty stomach and find out the food isn't prepared the way you need it to be.

Learn about the Foods You're Eating

Going on a candida diet is the perfect opportunity to read books on food and healing. Make time to spend a few afternoons at a bookstore, library, or health food store and browse through the books on health, cooking, and self-help. Many of these books will answer a lot of your questions about "why" (why me? why no sugar? why cook?). You also may meet a "healing friend" in the health section!

Start a Food/Mood Diary

This is a wonderful way to learn to listen to your body. You may think you're paying attention to everything you eat and how you feel afterward, but writing it all down and then looking back can put your food and moods in perspective.

Here's what to do:

First, find a blank notebook and answer the following questions:

- What were my moods like before candida?
- What moods do I experience now?
- What do I want my moods to be like five years from now?

Remember, moods can be *good* and bad.

Next, eat and then write down the foods you are eating. Fifteen minutes later record how you feel. You can write down a word to describe your feeling or draw a picture of how you feel. Anything that conveys your mood. If you cannot think of what mood you are in, write anything down, even if it's "I cannot think what mood I'm in!"

Be aware that you can have a delayed reaction to some foods. Record all mood swings that come throughout the day, even if they do not occur directly after eating.

After one week, look back at your food/mood entries and reflect on the initial three questions you answered. Which mood made you feel like question number 1, number 2, or number 3? Identify the food you ate to create that mood. Begin to eat more of the foods that put you in a better mood. Continue the diary until you feel you don't need or want it any more.

Do the Organic Carrot Experiment

I cannot stress enough the benefits of eating organic food. Foods sprayed with chemicals are not good for us, especially for a person with candida who already has an overload of toxins in his immune system. Washing vegetables well or peeling the skin off will not get rid of the chemicals, they are in the cell structures of the vegetables.

Organic vegetables and meats are not only healthier, but they taste better. Not convinced yet? Do the carrot experiment. Buy 2¼ pounds of organic carrots and 2¼ pounds of non-organic carrots and wash them well.

- Chop half of a non-organic carrot into strips and slowly, with your eyes closed, eat it raw. Record in three words how it tastes. Then do the same for the organic carrot. Compare your answers. Not convinced yet?

- Steam an organic and non-organic carrot. Do the same test as above. Not convinced yet?

- Make a quick carrot soup. Put two large carrots in a saucepan with water. Let them boil for 15–20 minutes. Process the carrots and cooking liquid in your food processor until you have a smooth and soupy mixture. Do this for both the organic and non-organic carrots. Then taste.

It's your choice whether to buy organic or not, but remember that it is not only putting the right food into the body that helps a sick person get healthy, it should also be of the best quality.

Enrolling the Support of Your Partner

Most candida practitioners agree that if you have a supportive partner you will heal quicker and it will be much easier to stay on your diet. A supportive partner accepts your ups and downs and helps you through the process of rebounding to good health. Most partners who are unsupportive are this way because they do not understand what you are going through.

Here's what you can do to enroll the support of your partner. Find a quiet time to sit down with your partner and talk about your feelings, both on a physical and emotional level. Put on soft, relaxing background music and keep the lights dim. Agree not to answer the phone during your conversation or allow any other interruptions.

Begin by telling your partner how you have been feeling, starting with when the candida-like symptoms began appearing. If you are getting panic attacks, tell him about these and describe an instance when you had one and how it made you feel. Or describe what it has been like to have pain in your stomach and bloating all the time. Then talk about your new candida diet and your hopes and fears about embarking on such a diet. Tell your partner what you need and expect during your time of healing. Thank your partner for listening to you.

It is very important to go through this exercise with your partner because your not feeling good affects him too. Neither of you should deny this. A partner can be more understanding, accepting your new diet, and even joining you on the diet once he has been told in a calm and loving way how you are feeling. Otherwise, as strange as this may seem, he may not know how you feel.

Meeting the Needs of Children with Candida

If you are a parent trying to get your child on a candida diet you could feel overwhelmed by the challenge of weaning them off processed foods and sugar. You can be successful in getting him to eat candida foods using patience, humor, and actively involving your child in the process. Here are a few suggestions:

- Slowly replace processed foods with candida foods. Replace sugar-laden cereals with those with no sugar; use soy milk instead of cow's milk.

- Prepare candida foods that are familiar in appearance. Cook tofu burgers, tofu hot dogs, baked potato chips, sweet potatoes.

- Include your child in the preparation of meals. Young children usually love to help. This may seem difficult if your child is older and unaccustomed to helping in the kitchen, or you feel you have little time to let him help, but it is very important. Let him grate carrots, wash vegetables, or clean beans. Most kids love to eat things they were involved in making.

- Pack popcorn, a socially acceptable snack, in her lunch so she has something to eat when other kids are munching on processed snacks. Of course, your child will inevitably eat with other kids and be tempted by their food, but if she has a nutritious snack with her at least she has an option not to eat her friends' food.

- Believe that your child can make the switch to candida foods and that his health will greatly improve. If you don't believe it will work, it probably won't. So many children have become healthier and their behavior, including signs of autism, markedly improved once they went on a candida diet.

Cheating   It is difficult to get better if you cheat a lot on this diet. The candida has to die and it cannot do so unless you starve it, which means not eating certain foods. Sometimes life circumstances make a new way of eating seem impossible. Respect your limits and know when it is the right time for you to start a strict candida diet. The sooner the better, but if you go on the diet and constantly cheat you only prolong the amount of time you will have to stay on the diet.

Candida sufferers who have been seriously ill for a long time rarely cheat because getting better feels like a matter of life or death for them. If you are not "deathly sick" you may be more tempted to cheat periodically. "This one chocolate bar won't hurt me." Think again! One chocolate bar could erase the hard work you put into staying on the diet up until that point. If you really want a piece of chocolate go ahead and have it, but eat only half of it and record how you feel afterward. Once you feel the connection between eating certain foods and feeling bad you probably won't cheat too many times. If you do not cheat the candida dies off and cravings for junk food often cease.

Will I Ever Get Off This Diet?

The first question most candida sufferers usually ask is, "Will I ever get off this diet?" and "When?" We have been conditioned by Western medicine to have an answer and a figure to go with that answer. It's okay to be told, "You have a bladder infection and it will clear up two weeks after you take this medicine" or "You have to have a back operation and won't be on your feet for six months to a year." But when you are told, "You need to create a diet with foods that suit your body, and how long it will take you to feel better depends on you," frightens many of us because the control is in your own hands.

Most people with candida who strictly adhere to the diet and receive proper nutritional treatment are able to come off the diet. The amount of time you will have to stay on the diet, however, depends on your body's needs. If you have been feeling bad for a very long time you may be on the diet for a couple of years. Others are off, at least the strict portion of the diet, in six months. Being on a candida diet is only one step in your healing process. It is a crucial step, but there are other aspects to feeling better that will determine how fast you get better. Many former candida sufferers find that over time their taste in foods change and they prefer eating a whole-food diet.

Pressuring yourself to know "Will I be on this diet for four months or eight months or a year or three years?" is pointless. You have an opportunity to take control of your own health, so commit yourself to being on a candida diet for however long it takes to feel better.

CHAPTER ELEVEN

Recipes to Please

Every day we need to eat, whether we like it or not. And every day we have to make choices about what to eat, whether we like it or not. I cannot stress enough that everyone is different. Candida sufferers, in particular, often have different food sensitivities. If the list of foods you cannot eat seems like it's five miles long right now, don't let that stop you from reading through the recipes in this chapter. You may find that many recipes are okay for you, but even if you don't, reading recipes is a great way to generate ideas about what to cook. You can prepare the same type of food using a grain, legume, or vegetable you can eat.

The recipes in this chapter use some ingredients you will be familiar with, and others you won't. Trying new foods can be an exciting way to make your diet more interesting, so please experiment. Aim to cook one dish a week that introduces a new ingredient. You may be amazed at how good new food can be.

All recipes are dairy-free and, of course, sugar- and yeast-free. Many are also gluten-free. Some people with candida might be able to eat more ingredients than those contained in these recipes. Deciding which ingredients are right for you is best done in consultation with your health practitioner, and by taking time to assess how your body is reacting and what it is telling you it wants (not what foods are delicious!).

Your adventure into healthy eating is about to begin, so take a deep breath and let's go!

BREAKFAST

You don't have time for breakfast? Set your alarm 15 minutes earlier and make time! This is a very important meal in your day, especially if you have low blood sugar, which is very common among candida sufferers. If you are pressed for time, at least sit down and eat a bowl of cereal (homemade muesli or another sugar-free cereal from the health food store) with soy milk or another non-dairy alternative. Your body will thank you.

The following recipes take between 10 to 20 minutes to prepare. If you start cooking them when you get up, by the time you have showered and dressed your breakfast will be ready.

All the breakfast recipes serve one person.

Hot Oatmeal

If you use organic oats, oatmeal tastes a lot better. It's just like you've added butter!

9 oz oats

17 oz filtered water

Put the oats and water in a pot and bring to a rapid boil. Turn off the heat, cover and let sit for 10–15 minutes.

Variations

Use soy milk instead of water for a richer taste.

Add toasted sunflower seeds for more flavor.

Hot Millet and Quinoa Cereal

Millet and quinoa are two wonderful gluten-free grains that you should get to know. This may sound like a strange combination, but it tastes surprisingly nice and is filling.

4½ oz millet

4½ oz quinoa

1¼ pints filtered water

Put the millet, quinoa, and water in a saucepan and bring to a boil. Turn down the heat and let simmer for 20 minutes. Blend everything together in a food processor until it looks smooth and creamy. Now it's ready.

Variations

Cook with a handful of linseeds.

Millet is a great, creamy cereal in its own right. Boil 9 oz of millet and one carrot in 1¾ pints water. Cook for 20 minutes, purée it and you have a sweet-tasting breakfast cereal.

Hot Sesame and Rice Cereal

If you feel your candida is not too severe, you can use rice left over from the night before. It will then only take 5 minutes to reheat instead of 40 minutes to cook.

7 oz brown rice

17 oz filtered water

Sesame seeds to taste

Bring the rice and water to a boil in a pot, then reduce the heat and simmer for 40 minutes. While the rice is cooking, or the night before, toast the sesame seeds in a dry pan over a high heat, turning frequently until they are toasted. Watch constantly as they burn easily. Leave them to cool, then store in an airtight jar. When the rice is done, blend until smooth. Add sesame seeds until the flavor is as you like it.

Variations

Use soy milk instead of water for a richer taste.

Add a grated carrot for sweetness.

Muesli

Muesli can be made with any combination of oats, millet flakes, brown rice flakes, barley flakes, nuts, and seeds. All of these ingredients can be bought in a health food store. Experimenting with ingredients that you are not sensitive to is the key.

1 lb oats

12 oz barley flakes

12 oz wheat flakes

6 oz brown rice flakes

a handful of sunflower seeds

a handful of coconut flakes

Combine 1 lb oats, 12 oz barley flakes, 12 oz wheat flakes, 6 oz brown rice flakes, a handful of sunflower seeds and coconut flakes.

For a gluten-free alternative, combine 12 oz millet flakes, 6 oz brown rice flakes, sesame seeds, and a nut and seed mixture to taste (grind the nuts and seeds up in a coffee grinder).

Scrambled Tofu

This takes 15 minutes to prepare.

1 teaspoon oil

½ onion, finely chopped

¼ teaspoon turmeric

½ carrot, grated

½ celery stick, finely chopped

4 oz tofu

Heat the oil in a pan. Sauté the onion and turmeric for 1 minute. Add the vegetables, beginning with the carrot, then the celery. Sauté for 3–5 minutes.

Crumble the tofu into a bowl, then add to the sautéed vegetables and stir. Cover and steam for 5 minutes, stirring occasionally.

Variations

Add some unfermented soy sauce at the end to give it a salty taste.

Add ginger or garlic.

Garnish with fresh parsley.

LUNCH

Baked Beans

This can be served over a baked potato, brown rice, or toasted yeast-free bread.

7 oz dried haricot beans

1¾ pints filtered water

1 large onion, diced

1 tablespoon olive oil

5 medium tomatoes, quartered

2 tablespoons tomato purée
   (make sure it contains no citric acid)

1 teaspoon paprika

freshly ground black pepper

Soak the haricot beans overnight. The next day, drain the beans and cook them for 1 hour in 1¾ pints fresh filtered water until soft. Sauté the onion in the oil for 1 minute.

Add the tomatoes, tomato purée, and paprika. Stir for 2–3 minutes until thick. Blend the tomato mixture in a food processor until smooth. Mix with the haricot beans, add pepper to taste, and warm through over a medium heat for a few minutes.

Root Vegetable Soup

If you don't feel like spending much time preparing lunch, this is the soup for you.

2 carrots

2 parsnips

1 onion

¼ rutabaga

1 tablespoon dried rosemary

1¾ pints filtered water

1 teaspoon ground ginger

Wash all the vegetables well, cut off the ends, put everything in a saucepan whole, add water to cover the vegetables, bring to a boil and then let simmer for 15–20 minutes. Drain, reserving the cooking water, and blend all the cooked vegetables in a food processor. Then add the reserved water until the mixture is smooth and soup-like.

Variations

For a heavier soup add olive oil.

You can use virtually any vegetable to make this soup. Also experiment with different mild spices, especially garlic and ginger.

Cream of Broccoli Soup

1 head of broccoli, chopped into large florets

1 potato

4 oz soy milk

Bring all the ingredients to a boil, then simmer, covered, for 15–10 minutes.

Purée, adding more soy milk if necessary.

Variations

If you cannot eat potatoes, use oats to thicken the soup. Mix in 3 oz of oats with the vegetables at the beginning, stirring frequently while the mixture is heating to a boil, then simmer for 15 minutes and purée.

If you are allergic to broccoli, substitute a vegetable that is okay for you.

Brown Rice Salad

This is a great dish to take to a summer afternoon party or pack for lunch. If you find you have some left over, blend in a food processor with some water and use it as a gravy.

7 oz brown rice

17 oz filtered water

1 medium carrot

½ head of broccoli, diced

1 small onion

¼ small cabbage, chopped

1 tablespoon chopped fresh parsley

2–3 tablespoons toasted sunflower seeds

Simmer the brown rice in the water, covered, for about 40 minutes. Meanwhile, boil the carrots, broccoli, and onion together for 2–3 minutes. Lift them out, drain, and let cool.

In the same boiling water, cook the cabbage for 1 minute. Drain and cool.

Mix all the cooked ingredients together with the rice and remaining ingredients in a bowl.

Variations

Use any vegetables you like or add cooked organic chicken for a chicken and rice salad.

You can poor the Lemon, Garlic, and Oil Dressing (see page 158) on top.

Quinoa Pilaf

This is a wonderful quick pilaf, very light and fluffy.

1¼ pints filtered water

9 oz quinoa

1 leek, finely chopped

1 carrot, grated

1 red onion, sliced

1 tablespoon fresh parsley, finely chopped

Heat the water in a pan. Add the quinoa and leek just before the water boils. Cover and simmer for 20 minutes. Turn off the heat and add the carrot, red onion, and parsley. Let sit covered for 5 minutes.

Variations

Substitute any grain you like instead of quinoa.

Put in cooked chickpeas for a nutty taste, or add toasted sesame seeds.

Workday Lunches

- *Baked potato*   Fill with candida-friendly foods, like a can of tuna. This is also great to order if you go out for a meal.

- *Sandwiches*   Flat breads, like any floured tortilla or chapati, make great bread alternatives. Yeast-free soda bread is another option. Fill your sandwich with hummus, avocados, sprouts, lettuce, tofu, beans—the possibilities are endless!

- *Salads*   Making a salad with different types of lettuce, adding sprouts and some toasted sunflower and pumpkin seeds is a great meal that travels well in a container. Bring along rice cakes and a spread (hummus or almond butter) and you have a meal.

- *Soups*   Most workplaces have facilities to reheat food. This is one of the few times I would say be flexible and use a microwave. Your food may be less nutritious, but you will have food in your stomach and be able to continue working. Make soup the night before and carry it in a container to work or see what soup the local take-out sells—vegetarian restaurants often have one vegan soup available on a daily basis. If they don't have a vegan selection ask them if they could offer it once a week. Many restaurants like to do this sort of thing to please their customers. Bring some oatcakes with you and your meal is complete.

- *Pasta salads*   There are lots of wheat-free pastas available. Health food stores carry rice pasta, corn pasta, and even millet pasta. Cook pasta the night before you want to take it for lunch. Lightly steam assorted vegetables (don't overcook vegetables —it lowers their nutritional content) and mix with the pasta. Refrigerate. Put Lemon, Garlic, and Oil Dressing (see page 158) on the pasta salad right before you're about to eat it so the salad isn't soaked in oil. This can also be a quick meal for dinner.

DINNER

Tofu Walnut Burgers

This is a great dish to serve to children.

7 oz brown rice

1¾ pints filtered water

1 onion, finely chopped

2 garlic cloves

1 carrot, grated

1 tablespoon olive oil

9 oz tofu

2 tablespoons unfermented soy sauce (optional)

2 organic eggs

2 oz walnuts

Preheat the oven to 400° F.

Simmer the rice in the water in a covered pan for 40 minutes. Sauté the onion, garlic, and carrot in the olive oil for 3–5 minutes. Place in a large mixing bowl. Then in a food processor, mix together the tofu, brown rice, and soy sauce if using, until it forms a thick, smooth consistency. Add this to sautéed vegetables, and mix well. Beat the two eggs and mix them in. Add the walnuts. Form round burgers and place on a floured baking sheet. Bake in the preheated oven for 45 minutes.

Variations

Substitute another nut for the walnuts.

Use a different grain instead of brown rice.

Vegetable Curry

1 onion, sliced

1 tablespoon fresh grated root ginger

1 tablespoon sesame oil

1 carrot, chopped

3 potatoes, chopped

1 small cauliflower, chopped

1 medium zucchini, chopped

1 teaspoon turmeric

1 teaspoon curry powder
(make sure it has no added sugar)

8 oz filtered water

Sauté the onion and ginger in the oil for 1 minute. Add the carrot and potatoes and cook for 2 minutes. Add the cauliflower, zucchini, and stir. Then stir in the turmeric and curry powder, coating the vegetables with the spices. Pour some filtered water into the mixture until the curry is the right consistency. Break up the potatoes and cover, simmering until the vegetables are tender.

Variations

Add cooked chickpeas or meat for a hearty meal or try cubes of tofu.

Add cashew nuts.

Use garlic instead of ginger—or both!

Use different vegetables (leave the potato, though as it makes for a great thick, saucy consistency).

Lentil Bake

8 oz red lentils, soaked overnight

17 oz filtered water

1 carrot, grated

1 parsnip, finely chopped

1 onion, finely chopped

5 tablespoons wholemeal flour

2 organic eggs

1 garlic clove

Preheat the oven to 400° F.

Cook the lentils in the water for 15–20 minutes until the water has been absorbed. In a bowl mix the cooked lentils with the remaining ingredients. Put the mixture in a floured one-pound loaf pan and bake in the preheated oven for 30 minutes.

Variations

If you're allergic to wholemeal flour use any flour you can eat. Alternatively, put in 7 oz of well-cooked brown rice instead of flour.

Use any mild spices you can tolerate.

Instead of baking, form the mixture into burgers, coat with flour, and cook for 20–25 minutes.

Tim's Shepherd's Pie

7 oz potatoes, chopped

1 large onion, chopped

4 oz soy margarine, unhydrogenated

1–2 tablespoons soy milk

2 carrots, sliced thinly

2 garlic cloves, crushed

9 oz ground lamb

4 oz butter beans, cooked

8 oz yeast-free vegetable stock

Preheat the oven to 400° F.

Boil the potatoes until they are soft. Meanwhile, gently cook the onions in all but 1½ oz of the margarine until they are soft. Drain the potatoes and put the remaining margarine and the soy milk in with the potatoes and mash until smooth. Add the carrots and garlic to the onions and cook for 1–2 minutes. Add the ground lamb, butter beans, and the vegetable stock. Cook for 20 minutes. Pour into a casserole dish and cover with the mashed potatoes. Bake in the preheated oven for 30 minutes or until the potatoes have browned nicely.

Variations

Use green lentils instead of ground lamb.

Use the bean of your choice.

Grate soy cheese on top for extra flavor.

If you are sensitive to potatoes substitute Millet "Mashed Potatoes" (see page 152).

Add any fresh herbs you like. Chopped rosemary is delicious in this dish.

Lemon Ginger Chicken

6 lemons

4 pieces organic chicken

1 tablespoon freshly grated root ginger

Preheat the oven to 400° F.

In a casserole dish, squeeze the juice of 3 of the lemons over the chicken. Thinly slice the other 3 lemons, leaving the rind on. Put the lemon slices over the chicken in the casserole dish. Grate the ginger and pour the juice from the ginger (including the grated bits) over the chicken. Bake in the preheated oven for 1½ hours.

Variations

Add mild fresh herbs.

Add a little soy milk and flour to the lemon juice to make a richer sauce.

Replace the ginger with garlic, or use both!

Vegetable and Millet Casserole

13 oz millet

1 carrot, sliced

1 onion, chopped

1 tablespoon dried rosemary

½ pint filtered water

7 oz tofu

4 tablespoons olive oil

2 garlic cloves, crushed

1½ lbs spinach

Preheat the oven to 400° F.

Combine the millet, carrot, onion, and rosemary in a casserole dish with the filtered water. Cover the casserole dish and bake in the preheated oven for 45 minutes. Meanwhile, cut the tofu into large, thin slices and lightly cook them in the olive oil. Remove them from the oil, drain on a paper towel to remove any excess oil and let cool. In the same pan, leaving only a little olive oil in the pan, lightly cook the garlic with the spinach for a few minutes until wilted. Add a little water to the pan during frying to prevent the spinach from burning. Place the spinach on the side until the casserole has cooked. The casserole is done when all the water has been absorbed. When done, take the casserole out of the oven, remove the cover, and place a layer of tofu on top and then the spinach. Return to the oven and bake for 5–7 minutes, uncovered. Then enjoy with Tahini Sauce (see page 157).

Variations

Steam sweet potatoes, mash them, and add it as the layer before the tofu once the casserole has baked.

Add any herbs or ginger, which is especially good.

VEGETABLE SIDE DISHES

Millet "Mashed Potatoes"

If you are sensitive to potatoes this is the dish for you. It tastes like mashed potatoes; you won't believe there are no potatoes in the recipe!

1¾ pints filtered water

9 oz millet

1 small cauliflower

Bring the water to a boil, add the millet and cauliflower, cover and simmer for 25 minutes. Blend in a food processor, adding water if necessary to achieve the consistency of mashed potatoes.

Variations

You could use potatoes instead of cauliflower if you can eat them (use 4 potatoes, peeled and diced).

Add any herbs.

Add a little soy milk and soy margarine.

Add 4 fl oz soy milk mixed with 2 tablespoons tahini for a richer flavor.

Baked Potato Chips

3-4 medium potatoes, cut into chip shapes

1 tablespoon oil

Preheat the oven to 400° F.

In a bowl, coat the chips with the oil. Put them on a baking sheet in a single layer. Bake in the preheated oven for 35–40 minutes. Turn the chips several times while baking so they cook and brown evenly.

Variations

Use sweet potatoes instead of white potatoes. Not only do sweet potatoes have a wonderful natural flavor, but very few people have allergic reactions to sweet potatoes. Check them after 25 minutes because they usually take less time to cook than white potatoes.

Brussels Sprouts with Chestnuts

This is a wonderful, rich dish.

12 oz chestnuts in their shells

filtered water as required

2 tablespoons unhydrogenated soy margarine

1 lb 2 oz Brussels sprouts

Boil the chestnuts, unpeeled, in just enough water to cover until the shells feel soft and loose (about 10 minutes). Take the shells off the chestnuts. Warm the soy margarine in a pan, add the Brussels sprouts, and cook for 10 minutes. Add the chestnuts, stir, and cook for another 5 minutes or until the Brussels sprouts are cooked.

Variations

If you are able to include some fruit in your diet, try green grapes instead of or in addition to the chestnuts.

Use oil instead of soy margarine.

Nori Rolls

This dish impresses everyone. It looks like sushi and tastes great. You can take it to a party, sliced, or take it whole for lunch. Once you get the hang of it, it's very easy to make.

filtered water, as required

½ carrot, cut in thin strips

3 broccoli florets, cut into strips

1 spring onion, halved lengthways

1 sheet of nori (dried seaweed,
   available from groceries or health food stores)

7 oz cooked, cooled brown rice

4 oz toasted sesame seeds

Boil the water and cook the vegetables in it for 1–2 minutes. Then, drain the vegetables and let them cool. Place the nori on a flat surface. Spoon the rice onto the nori. Wet your fingers and press the rice evenly, very flat, over three quarters of the nori, leaving the quarter along the top edge empty. About 1 inch up from the bottom edge of the nori, sprinkle 1 teaspoon of the sesame seeds along in a line. Then lay out each vegetable lengthwise, one at a time, in strips on top of the sesame seeds. Lift the nori from the bottom and roll it up tightly and evenly, pressing the edge inward. Moisten the uncovered edge of the nori with water so it will stick to the roll to seal it. Allow to rest a few minutes. Cut into 1-inch slices, wiping the knife clean after each slice.

Variations

Use any vegetables, but choose ones of different colors if you can so it looks nice when you slice it.

Dip the slices in unfermented soy sauce to add extra flavor when eating.

SAUCES, DIPS, SPREADS & STUFFING

Tahini Sauce

4 oz tahini

1 teaspoon sesame oil

filtered water as required

Stir the tahini in a pan over a medium heat until it is lightly roasted. Add the oil. Stir in enough water in to achieve a sauce-like consistency. Simmer for 5 minutes. Do not let it boil because the tahini will curdle.

Variations

Add crushed garlic.

Sauté an onion until soft and add it to the sauce.

Lemon, Garlic, and Oil Dressing

4 oz olive oil

juice of ½ a lemon

1 garlic clove

In a small screw-top jar mix the olive oil and lemon juice. Add the garlic, leaving the clove whole. Shake and let sit for 5 minutes. If you put it in the refrigerator it will keep for a couple of days.

Variations

Use a different oil.

Add fresh herbs.

Don't use garlic, or add chopped parsley to counteract the garlic taste in your mouth (if you add parsley, use the dressing right away; it does not keep well).

Avocado and Tofu Spread

1 ripe avocado, stoned, and flesh scooped from skin

7 oz tofu

juice of 1 lemon

filtered water as required

Mash the avocado flesh with the tofu in a bowl. Add the lemon juice and mix well. Blend in food processor until smooth, adding water if necessary.

Variations

Add more water to make a sauce, less if you want a spread.

Throw in a clove of garlic to give it extra zing.

Hummus

Hummus is excellent for any occasion—as a dip for parties or spread in a sandwich. Plus, it's full of protein.

14 oz dried chickpeas

3½ pints filtered water

juice of 2 lemons

2 oz olive oil

3 garlic cloves

4 oz tahini

filtered water as required

Soak the chickpeas in water overnight. The next day, simmer the chickpeas in the filtered water for 1–2 hours, until they are soft. Let cool. Put all the ingredients, except the tahini and water, into a food processor and purée. Then add the tahini. Add water, if necessary, to create a smooth consistency.

Variations

Don't be afraid to add more of the main ingredients to make the hummus taste how you like it.

Add fresh herbs.

Use an avocado to make Avocado Hummus.

You can replace the chickpeas with tofu and create a Tofu Hummus.

White Sauce

2 tablespoons soy margarine

2-3 tablespoons flour

1¼ pints soy milk

In a pan, melt the soy margarine. Remove the pan from the heat, add the flour and mix into a smooth paste. Add the soy milk slowly, stirring frequently. Keep stirring while you bring the mixture to a boil, then simmer for 2–3 minutes. Add more soy milk, if necessary, to achieve a smooth consistency.

Variations

Add fresh herbs.

Replace the soy milk with a different type of milk, such as oat or rice.

Creamy Leek Sauce

2–3 leeks, chopped into ½-inch thick slices

3 teaspoons olive oil

filtered water as required

Steam the leeks for 10–12 minutes until soft. Transfer the slices to a food processor, add the olive oil, 2 tablespoons of water and purée for 1 minute. Add more water, if necessary, until you have a smooth sauce consistency.

Variations

Add herbs.

Add garlic.

Mix in soy milk instead of water.

Baked Garlic

For garlic lovers only! After you bake garlic it spreads like butter so use it on yeast-free breads or vegetables.

4 garlic cloves

2–3 teaspoons olive oil

4 oz filtered water

Preheat the oven to 400° F.

Remove the outer papery skin of the garlic and trim off the ends. Place the whole cloves of garlic in a baking dish. Pour the olive oil over them. Cover and bake in the preheated oven for 20 minutes. Add the water and baste the garlic, then continue to bake covered for 1 hour until the garlic is very soft when pierced with a fork.

Variations

Add any herbs and freshly ground black pepper.

Brown Rice Stuffing

14 oz brown rice

½ pint filtered water

1 large onion

1 garlic clove

1 tablespoon oil

4 tablespoons filtered water

1 yeast-free vegetable stock cube

7 oz chestnuts

parsley, chopped

Preheat the oven to 400° F.

Simmer the brown rice in the water, covered, for 40 minutes. Sauté the onion and garlic in the oil until soft. Pour in the water, dissolve the vegetable stock cube in it and simmer for 2 minutes. Take the chestnuts out of their shells (boil them until soft and then the shells will come off easily), chop and mix them in a bowl with all the other ingredients. Purée in a food processor—the consistency should be like stuffing. Bake in an oiled baking dish, covered, in the preheated oven for 30 minutes or use to stuff a chicken and cook for the time and the temperature that is right for its size.

Variations

You can change any of the ingredients to make a savory stuffing.

Replace the brown rice with a different grain (couscous or millet).

Add any herbs you like.

Choose a different nut (walnuts or pine nuts) if you don't like chestnuts.

Add more oil for an extra moist taste.

YEAST-FREE BREADS

Tortillas

These are great fresh, used to make a sandwich, or make a lot on a day you have extra time and freeze them—they'll reheat in the oven in less than five minutes.

6 oz flour

4 oz filtered water

1 teaspoon sunflower oil

Mix the flour, water, and oil together until the dough clumps together in a ball. Break off small balls of dough, and on a floured board knead until soft. Then one at a time, roll out the ball of dough with a rolling pin until it is like a pancake. Flour both sides of the tortilla and bake in a hot pan, about 3 minutes on each side (you do not need oil in the pan).

Variations

Experiment with different flours.

Coconut Bread

This is delicious fresh and also freezes well.

5 oz desiccated coconut

11 oz wholemeal flour

12 oz warm filtered water

1 teaspoon sunflower oil

Mix the coconut and flour in a bowl and make a well in the center. Add the warm water and mix gently. Heat the oil in a pan, distributing the oil evenly. Drop 4 or 5 heaping tablespoons of the batter into the hot pan, leaving adequate space between each spoonful. Flatten each one with a spatula until it is no more than 3 inches in diameter and ¼ inch thick, and cook for 3–4 minutes until brown on the bottom. Turn them over and cook 3–4 minutes longer. Let cool. Repeat with the remaining batter.

Variations
Use soy margarine instead of oil.
Try soy milk instead of water.

DESSERTS

Carrot Pudding

14 oz carrots, grated

1¼ pints soy milk

1 teaspoon grated fresh root ginger

1 teaspoon sunflower oil

In a pan mix the carrots, soy milk, and ginger; cover and simmer over a very low heat for 1–1½ hours, stirring occasionally until the liquid evaporates. Then in a clean pan heat the oil and spoon in the carrot mixture, sautéeing it. The mixture is wet, but will dry out as you sauté. Stir continually to prevent it from sticking. Cook for 5–10 minutes. Spoon into a serving dish.

Variations

If your candida isn't too bad, add raisins or walnuts.

Baked Apples

This is a treat you can eat when you feel better.

4–6 apples

5 oz raisins

4 oz walnuts

2 tablespoons tahini

juice of 1 lemon

Preheat the oven to 350° F.

Core the apples and pierce with a fork to prevent the skins from bursting during cooking. Place the apples in a baking dish. Mix the raisins, walnuts, tahini, and lemon in a bowl. Spoon the filling into the center of the apples. Cover with foil and bake for 30 minutes. They're ready when you can pierce them easily with a fork.

Variations

Add vanilla, if you can tolerate it.

Use some ginger.

Substitute any dried fruit or nuts for the raisins and walnuts.

Eliminate all dried fruit and nuts and fill the apples only with tahini.

Sesame Oatcakes

11 oz oat flour

4 oz toasted sesame seeds

3 oz olive oil

1 teaspoon sesame oil

3 oz filtered water

Preheat the oven to 325° F.

Mix the flour and seeds together. Stir in both the oils and water. Mix thoroughly. Roll out on a baking sheet with oiled wax paper laid over the dough. Cut into squares with a knife. Bake for 10–12 minutes until lightly brown.

Variations

Use any flour instead of oat flour.

Eliminate the sesame seeds and you have plain oatcakes!

Snacks

Here are a few ideas for delicious snacks.

- *Toasted sunflower and pumpkin seeds*   In a dry pan, cook some seeds over a medium-high heat, stirring until they smell toasted. Let cool.

- *Popcorn*   If you are not allergic to corn this is a great snack. Do not use microwave popcorn. You can pop your own by putting 1 tablespoon of oil and 7 oz of corn kernels in a heavy bottomed pan, covering the pan, and cooking over a high heat, shaking it periodically and making sure some air is allowed to escape. The popcorn is ready when the popcorn stops popping.

- *Brown rice cakes*   Or any other grain rice cake. These are available in health food stores and many groceries.

- *Raw vegetable sticks*   These are great to bring to work or eat at home, dipping them into hummus.

- *Oatcakes*   Buy only those that have no added malt.

- *Potato and corn chips*   You can eat small amounts of any brands without artificial flavorings.

QUICK MEALS

If you want a nutritious meal in a hurry try:

- Root Vegetable Soup and Tortillas (see pages 139 and 166)
- salad with Tahini Sauce (see page 157)
- couscous cooked with assorted vegetables (ask in your health food store for gluten-free couscous)
- pan-fried fish with steamed vegetables
- pasta, steamed vegetables, and Lemon, Garlic, and Oil Dressing (see page 158)
- canned tuna with pasta or brown rice and vegetables

Keep your kitchen stocked with these nutritious foods for when you have little time or just don't feel like cooking. On days when you have more time, cook beans, freeze them, and use them later during the week when time is short. Freezing food for no more than two weeks is okay. However, do not reheat the food in a microwave.

Cooking for
Special Times

You can incorporate the candida foods into your daily life and have fun, too. Once you gain some confidence with your cooking, try preparing candida foods for different occasions.

Special Holidays

You *can* get through special holidays on your new diet! Try the following menu, using the recipes mentioned in this chapter.

- Lemon Ginger Chicken or Lentil Bake (see pages 149 and 147)
- Brussels Sprouts with Chestnuts (see page 154)
- Roast potatoes, parsnips, and carrots
- Brown Rice Stuffing (see page 164)
- Tahini Sauce (see page 157)
- Baked Apples (see page 170)

Candida Dinner Parties

As mentioned in Chapter Ten, having a candida dinner party can be a great way to introduce hesitant family and friends to your new foods. Here is a sample menu using recipes from this chapter.

PRE-DINNER SNACKS:

Toasted Sunflower and Pumpkin Seeds (see page 172)

Nori Rolls (see page 155)

MAIN MEAL:

Lemon Ginger Chicken (see page 149)

Creamy Leek Sauce (see page 162)

Millet "Mashed Potatoes" (see page 152)

Steamed Greens and Carrots

DESSERT

Carrot Pudding (see page 169)

Theme Meals

A theme meal combines your candida foods with a special focus to lighten the atmosphere. Here are a few menu suggestions for the theme meals mentioned in Chapter Ten.

MEXICAN NIGHT

- Baked beans (see page 138)
- Tortillas (see page 166)
- Brown rice
- Shredded lettuce and grated carrots
- Sprouts
- Soy cheese

YANKEE NIGHT

- Tofu Walnut Burgers (use yeast-free soda bread as a bun!) (see page 145
- Baked Potato Chips (see page 153)
- Assorted steamed vegetables

PICNIC NIGHT

- Root Vegetable Soup (see page 139)
- Hummus (see page 160)
- Brown Rice Salad (see page 141)
- Raw vegetable sticks
- Rice cakes

APPENDIX

Quick List of Alternative Foods

Keep this list on the refrigerator to remind you that there are foods you can buy that are similar to the foods you used to eat. You may not be familiar with some of the foods, but they are all available in good health food stores. When you shop, carefully read the ingredients of the foods you buy to make sure you can eat them. Add any new foods to this list that you discover.

Cold Breakfast Cereals

- Puffed brown rice
- Brown rice or millet flakes
- Kashi puffed multigrain cereal
- Shredded Wheat
- Unsweetened cornflakes

Bread

- Tortillas, chapatis (not those made with white flour)
- Yeast-free wholemeal soda bread
- Rice cakes
- Oatcakes (only the unsweetened ones)
- Yeast-free pumpernickel bread

Milk

- Unsweetened soy milk

- Oat milk

- Coconut milk

- Brown rice milk

Butter

- Dairy-free. Unhydrogenated margarines

- Almond, cashew, and hazelnut butters (not peanut butter; it can carry mold)

Sugar

- Fruits

- Use apple juice to sweeten anything

- Brown rice syrup

- Fruit-only jams

Note: For at least the first few months everyone with candida should avoid all sugars. After this time some people can slowly reintroduce sugar. When you are ready to reintroduce some sugar, it is best to try unrefined sugars.

Refined Carbohydrates

These are white flour, white rice, and so on.

- Whole grains, like brown rice, millet, barley, bulgar wheat, quinoa, spelt, kamut, amaranth, corn

- Potatoes

- Whole grain pastas

Wheat and gluten

- Brown rice, millet, quinoa, spelt, kamut, amaranth, corn

- Pastas using the grains above

- Gluten-free products that do not contain ingredients you cannot eat (like sugar)

Non-organic Meats, Poultry, and Fish

- Free-range and organic meat and poultry
- Free-range and organic eggs
- Canned tuna
- Beans and legumes
- Tofu

Food Elimination and Symptom Chart

IF YOU ELIMINATE:

sugar, coffee, alcohol, milk and milk products, meats, fats, protein

YOU MAY FEEL . . .

tiredness, drowsiness, depression, feelings of alienation, lack of coordination, headaches, shakiness, nervousness, tension, inability to relax, excess mucus (possibly manifesting as sinus problems), acne, temporary cysts, foul body odor, coated tongue, feelings of being toxic, skin eruptions

FOR . . .

1–5 days

1–10 days

9–5 days or more, depending on the extent of the drinking

starting up to 3 months after the food was stopped and then for a year or two

varies: 1–4 weeks with a fast, 6–10 months for the deeper accumulations

This gives you an idea of physical symptoms that may occur when you eliminate different foods from your diet. You will not necessarily experience every symptom on the list; most symptoms are a sign of healing and will go away when the body becomes strong again. If your symptoms persist for an unusually long period of time, or just don't feel right, see your health practitioner.

Source: Annemarie Colbin, *Food and Healing*

Common Symptoms that Indicate You May Have Allergies

Reviewing your medical history from infancy to adulthood is an excellent way to get a complete picture of your health and identify allergies. Read through the list below and check off which symptoms apply to you. These symptoms are often present when you have allergies to food or something in the environment. Even if you check off just a few symptoms below and you feel bad, you should contact a qualified health practitioner for diagnosis and advice.

Symptoms in infancy and childhood

Colic as an infant

Difficulty gaining weight

Skin rashes

Frequent illnesses

Difficulty sleeping

Traditionally recognized allergic reactions (asthma, hives, etc.)

Earaches or fluid in the ears

Swollen glands

Pale face

Behavioral problems

Bedwetting (after age of 3)

Short attention span

Runny or stuffy nose

Coughing or wheezing

Muscle aches

"Growing pains"

Constipation

Diarrhea

Dark circles under the eyes

Puffiness under the eyes

Glassy eyes after eating

Sore throat

Stomach aches

Headaches

Learning disabilities

Hyperactivity

Symptoms in adulthood

Physical symptoms

Digestive problems—gas, bloating, belching

Abdominal distension

Sore throat

Phlegm in throat

Coughing or wheezing

Sneezing

Rapid heartbeat after eating

Heart palpitations after eating

Muscle aches

Joint pain

Dark circles, bags, or puffiness under the eyes

Red earlobes after eating

Watery eyes

"Sand" in the eyes

Stomach aches

Constipation and diarrhea

Rectal itching

Stuffy or runny nose

Sinus problems

Headaches

Loss of physical coordination

Swollen joints

Difficulty urinating

Water retention

Emotional symptoms

Fatigue

Drowsiness

Insomnia

Irritability

Mood swings

Depression

Crying

Anxiety

Paranoia

Schizophrenic behavior

Tendency to get angry easily

Nervousness

Loss of memory

Difficulty concentrating

Symptoms related to eating

Compulsive eating

Certain foods improve mood

Bingeing

Feeling better or worse after eating

Craving specific foods, such as bread, ice cream

Addiction to alcohol or drugs

Feeling strong aversion to certain foods

Family history

One or both parents having the symptoms above

Family members who experience any traditional allergies

Source: Gary Null, *Good Food, Good Mood*

Useful Addresses

Food Allergies and Food Intolerance

American Academy of Environmental Medicine (AAEM)
7701 East Kellogg Avenue, Suite 625
Wichita, KS 67207
phone: 316-684-5500
fax: 316-684-5709
web site: www.aaem.com

American EPD Society
P.O. Box 31126
Santa Fe, NM 87594-1126
phone: 505-984-0004

Colonic Irrigation

International Association for Colon Hydrotherapy
P.O. Box 461285
San Antonio, TX 78246-1285
phone: 210-366-2888
fax: 210-366-2999
web site: www.i-act.org

Myalgic Encephalomyelitis (ME)
or Chronic Fatigue Syndrome Organizations

**Chronic Fatigue and Immune Dysfunction Syndrome
Association of America**
P.O. Box 220398
Charlotte, NC 28222
fax: 704-365-2343
phone: 800-442-3437
web site: www.cfids.org

National Chronic Fatigue Syndrome and Fibromyalgia Association
P.O. Box 18426
Kansas City, MO 64133
phone: 816-313-2000

American Association for Chronic Fatigue Syndrome
c/o Harborview Medical Center
325 Ninth Avenue
Box 359780
Seattle, WA 98104
phone: 206-521-1932
fax: 206-521-1930
web site: www.aacfs.org

Products

BioCare
54 Northfield Road
Norton
Birmingham B 30 IJ

Further Reading

Astor, Stephen, et al. *Hidden Food Allergies: Finding the Foods That Cause You Problems and Removing Them from Your Diet* (Avery, 1997).

Chopich, Erika J. *Healing Your Aloneness* (Harper SanFrancisco, 1990).

Crook, William G., et al. *Chronic Fatigue Syndrome and the Yeast Connection: A Get-Well Guide for People with This Often Misunderstood Illness—And Those Who Care for Them* (Professional Books, 1992).

Demitrack, Mark A., et al. *Chronic Fatigue Syndrome: An Integrative Approach to Evaluation and Treatment* (Guilford Press, 1996).

Diamond, Harvey and Marilyn. *Fit For Life* (Warner Books, 1987).

Evennett, Karen. *Garlic: The Natural Remedy* (Ulysses Press, 1998).

Fulder, Stephen. *Garlic: Nature's Original Remedy* (Inner Traditions, 1999).

Goldberg, Burton. *Alternative Medicine Guide to Chronic Fatigue, Fibromyalgia and Environmental Illness* (Future Medicine Publishing, 1998).

Greenwood, Sadja. *Menopause, Naturally: Preparing for the Second Half of Life* (Volcano Press, 1996).

Hayes, Alan. *It's So Natural House Book* (HarperCollins Australia, 1998).

Hill, Clare. *The Ancient and Healing Art of Aromatherapy* (Ulysses Press, 1998).

Hunt, Jennifer. *Irritable Bladder & Incontinence: A Natural Approach* (Ulysses Press, 1998).

McGrath, Mike, ed. *The Best of Organic Gardening: Over 50 Years of Organic Advice and Reader-Proven Techniques from America's Best-Loved Gardening Magazine* (Rodale Press, 1996).

Natelson, Benjamin H. *Facing and Fighting Fatigue: A Practical Approach* (Yale University Press, 1998).

Naylor, Nicola. *Discover Essential Oils* (Ulysses Press, 1998).

Peck, M. Scott. *The Road Less Traveled* (Simon & Schuster, 1998).

Selby, Anna. *New Again! The 28-Day Detox Plan for Body and Soul* (Ulysses Press, 1999).

Trickett, Shirley. *Anxiety & Depression: A Natural Approach* (Ulysses Press, 1997).

Trickett, Shirley. *Irritable Bowel Syndrome & Diverticulosis: A Self-Help Plan* (Thorsons, 1992).

Yepsen, Roger, ed. *1,001 Old-Time Garden Tips: Timeless Bits of Wisdom on How to Grow Everything Organically, from the Good Old Days When Everyone Did* (Rodale Press, 1998).

Bibliography

Adverse Drug Reaction Bulletin, no. 121 (December 1986).

Becker, Robert O. *The Body Electric: Electromagnetism and the Foundation of Life* (William Morrow & Co., 1987).

British Journal of Dermatology, vol. 123 (1990), 319–323.

"Candida Peritonitis and Cimetidine," *The Lancet* (September 30, 1978).

"Candidiasis: Current Misconceptions," *CMAJ*, vol. 139 (October 1988).

Chopra, Deepak. *Creating Health: How to Wake Up the Body's Intelligence* (Houghton Mifflin, 1995).

Colbin, Annemarie. *Food and Healing* (Ballantine Books, 1996).

Cummings, John H. "Short-Chain Fatty Acids in the Human Colon," *Gut*, vol. 22 (1981), 76–79.

Eaton, K. K. "Gut Fermentation: A Reappraisal of the Old Clinical Condition with Diagnostic Tests and Management: Discussion Paper," *Journal of the Royal Society of Medicine*, vol. 84 (November 1991).

Hilton, Al and Warnock, D. W. *British Journal of Obstetrics* (1975), 922–926.

"Invasive Candidiasis Following Cimetidine Therapy," *American Journal of Gastroenterology*, vol. 1 (1988), 102–103.

H. R. Jenkins, et al. "Food Allergy: The Major Cause of Infantile Colitis," *Annals of Allergy*, vol. 153 (October 1984).

Kreiger, Dolores. *Therapeutic Touch: How To Use Your Hands to Help or Heal* (Simon & Schuster, 1992).

Macrae, Janet. *Therapeutic Touch: A Practical Guide* (Knopf, 1988).

Minney, S. "Garlic—The Forgotten Aid to Modern Medicine," *Biomed Newsletter*, vol. 1, no. 7 (1990).

Minney, S. "Investigation of Anticandidal Activity of Calcium and Magnesium Caprylate," *Biomed Research* (July 1992).

Neesby, T. "Butyric Acid Complexes: A New Approach to Food Intolerances," *Biomed Newsletter*, vol. 1, no. 2 (February 1990).

Null, Gary. *Good Food, Good Mood: Treating your Hidden Allergies* (St. Martin's Press, 1992).

Pfeiffer, Carl C. *Mental and Elemental Nutrients* (Keats Publishing, 1975).

Spellacy, W. N. "A Review of Carbohydrate Metabolism and the Oral Contraceptives," *American Journal of Obstetric Gynecology*, vol. 104 (1969), 448–60.

Swords, G. and Hunter, C. L. K. "Composition of Australian Tea Tree Oil (Melaleuca alternifolia)," *Journal of Agricultural Food and Chemistry*, vol. 26, no. 3 (1978).

Turner, Kristina. *Self-healing Cookbook* (Earthtones, 1989).

"Urinary Tract Infection and the Potential for a Natural Prophylactic Treatment," *Biomed Newsletter*, vol. 2, no. 8 (1991).

Werbach, Melvyn R. M.D. *Nutritional Influences on Illness* (Thorsons 1987).

Index

Ulysses Press Health Books

A Natural Approach Books

Written in a friendly, nontechnical style, *A Natural Approach* books address specific health issues and show you how to take an active part in your own treatment. Whether you suffer from panic attacks, endometriosis or depression, each book will provide you with a thorough understanding of your condition and detail organic solutions that offer immediate relief for your symptoms and effectively remedy their underlying causes.

Believing that disease is more than a combination of symptoms, these books offer integrated mind/body programs that take a positive, preventative approach. Since traditional drug therapy is not always the best solution (and can sometimes be the problem), these guides show how to use alternative treatments to supplement or replace conventional medicine.

ANXIETY & DEPRESSION
ISBN 1-56975-118-8, 144 pp, $9.95

CANDIDA
ISBN 1-56975-153-6, 208 pp, $11.95

ENDOMETRIOSIS
ISBN 1-56975-088-2, 184 pp, $9.95

FREE YOURSELF FROM TRANQUILIZERS
& SLEEPING PILLS
ISBN 1-56975-074-2, 192 pp, $9.95

IRRITABLE BLADDER & INCONTINENCE
ISBN 1-56975-089-0, 112 pp, $8.95

IRRITABLE BOWEL SYNDROME
2nd edition, ISBN 1-56975-188-9,
256 pp, $13.95

MIGRAINES
ISBN 1-56975-140-4, 240 pp, $10.95

PANIC ATTACKS
2nd edition, ISBN 1-56975-187-0,
156 pp, $9.95

The Natural Remedy Books

As home remedies and alternative treatments become increasingly accepted into the medical mainstream, people want information—not just hype and unproven claims—about the remedies they see in health food stores. *The Natural Remedy* books detail how these natural remedies have been used throughout history and how to safely incorporate them into an overall plan for maintaining good health.

CIDER VINEGAR
ISBN 1-56975-141-2, 144 pp, $8.95

GARLIC
ISBN 1-56975-097-1, 152 pp, $9.95

Discover Handbooks

Easy to follow and authoritative, *Discover* handbooks reveal an array of alternative therapies from around the world and demonstrate how to incorporate them into a program of good health.

Each book opens with information on the history and principles of the particular technique, then presents practical and straightforward guidance on ways in which it can be applied. Offering the tools needed to achieve and maintain an optimal state of health, the approach is one of personal improvement and self-reliance. Each of the books features: an introduction to the discipline; an explanation of its philosophy; step-by-step guide to its implementation; clear diagrams and charts; and case studies.

DISCOVER AYURVEDA
ISBN 1-56975-081-5, 128 pp, $8.95

DISCOVER COLOR THERAPY
ISBN 1-56975-093-9, 144 pp, $8.95

DISCOVER ESSENTIAL OILS
ISBN 1-56975-080-7, 128 pp, $8.95

DISCOVER MEDITATION
ISBN 1-56975-113-7, 144 pp, $8.95

DISCOVER NUTRITIONAL THERAPY
ISBN 1-56975-135-8, 120 pp, $8.95

DISCOVER OSTEOPATHY
ISBN 1-56975-115-3, 132 pp, $8.95

DISCOVER REFLEXOLOGY
ISBN 1-56975-112-9, 132 pp, $8.95

DISCOVER SHIATSU
ISBN 1-56975-082-3, 128 pp, $8.95

The Ancient and Healing Arts Books

The Ancient and Healing Arts books recount the development of healing art forms that have been used for thousands of years. Beautifully illustrated with full color on every page, they discuss the benefits of these time-honored techniques and offer detailed instructions on their use.

THE ANCIENT AND HEALING ART OF
AROMATHERAPY
ISBN 1-56975-094-7, 96 pp, $14.95

THE ANCIENT AND HEALING ART OF
CHINESE HERBALISM
ISBN 1-56975-139-0, 96 pp, $14.95

Other Health Titles

THE BOOK OF KOMBUCHA
ISBN 1-56975-049-1, 160 pp, $11.95
Explains the benefits of and addresses concerns about Kombucha, the widely used Chinese "tea mushroom."

HEALING REIKI: REUNITE MIND, BODY AND SPIRIT WITH HEALING ENERGY
ISBN 1-56975-162-5, 128 pp, $16.95

Examines the meaning, attitudes and history of Reiki while providing practical tips for receiving and giving this universal life energy.

HEPATITIS C: A PERSONAL GUIDE TO GOOD HEALTH
2nd edition, ISBN 1-56975-183-8, 180 pp, $13.95
Identifies the causes and symptoms of hepatitis C and presents conventional and alternative treatments for coping with the disease.

KNOW YOUR BODY: THE ATLAS OF ANATOMY
2nd edition, ISBN 1-56975-166-8, 160 pp, $12.95
Provides a a comprehensive, full-color guide to the human body.

MOOD FOODS
ISBN 1-56975-023-8, 192 pp, $11.95
Shows how the foods you eat influence your emotions and behavior.

NEW AGAIN!: THE 28-DAY DETOX PLAN FOR BODY AND SOUL
ISBN 1-56975-190-0, 128 pp, $16.95
Allows you to free your body *and* mind from toxins and live a healthy and balanced life.

THE 7 HEALING CHAKRAS: UNLOCKING YOUR BODY'S ENERGY CENTERS
ISBN 1-56975-168-4, 240 pp, $14.95
Explores the essence of chakras, vortices of energy that connect the physical body with the spiritual.

SEX HERBS: NATURE'S SEXUAL ENHANCERS
ISBN 1-56975-185-4, 140 pp, $12.95
Presents detailed descriptions of safe, natural products that boost sexual desire and pleasure.

YOUR NATURAL PREGNANCY: A GUIDE TO COMPLEMENTARY THERAPIES
ISBN 1-56975-059-9, 240 pp, $16.95
Details alternative therapies ranging from aromatherapy to yoga that can benefit pregnant women.

To order these books call 800-377-2542, fax 510-601-8307 or write to Ulysses Press, P.O. Box 3440, Berkeley, CA 94703-3440. All retail orders are shipped free of charge. California residents must include sales tax. Allow two to three weeks for delivery.

About the Author

Shirley Trickett trained as a nurse before becoming a counselor and teacher. She is based in the northeast of England and travels both throughout the United Kingdom and abroad with her work. She has worked with anxious and depressed people for several years, and is the author of *Free Yourself from Tranquilizers and Sleeping Pills* (Ulysses Press, 1997), *Anxiety & Depression: A Natural Approach* (Ulysses Press, 1997), *Headaches and Migraine* (Penguin, 1996), *Recipes for Health: Candida Albicans Yeast-Free and Sugar-Free Recipes* (Thorsons, 1994), and *The Irritable Bowel Syndrome and Diverticulosis* (Thorsons, 1990). In 1987 she won a Whitbread Community Care Award for her work.